# COLORADO

## JOURNEY GUIDE

### A DRIVING & HIKING GUIDE TO RUINS, ROCK ART, FOSSILS & FORMATIONS

WRITTEN BY JON KRAMER AND JULIE MARTINEZ
ILLUSTRATIONS BY VERNON MORRIS

Adventure Publications, Inc.
Cambridge, MN

## Authors' Dedications

To my fellow adventurer, life companion, and beautiful wife, Julie, whose gentle nature and thoughtful insights inspire me daily. Words cannot express . . .

–JON KRAMER

To my fellow adventurer, soul mate, and wonderful husband, Jon, whose love and support is always with me as we travel through life together and to my loving parents who instilled in me a sense of curiosity and profound love for the Natural World.

–JULIE MARTINEZ

To the ancient people who built and inhabited the ruins, pecked their artwork into stone, and scouted the trails we follow today

–VERN MORRIS

The authors would like to express gratitude and special thanks to those who treat the Earth and all its creatures with the reverence and respect they deserve. The Great Spirit smiles upon you each sunrise.

Photo credits by artist and page number:
**Cover photos by Jon Kramer and Julie Martinez**: Painted Hands Puelbo (main photo), Deer Creek Petroglyphs (left inset), Garden of the Gods (middle inset), Tyrannosaurus Rex skull (right inset)
**All photos copyright Jon Kramer and Julie Martinez unless otherwise noted.**
**Joyce Alexander:** 48 **Mike Blakeman:** 206, 208 (both), 209 **Glenwood Hot Springs Lodge and Pool:** 101 (both) **David Harris/courtesy of Glenwood Caverns Adventure Park:** 98 **Bernadette Heath:** 200 (bottom) **Richard Johnson:** 66, 67, 68, 69 **Mesa Verde Country®:** 198 **Wendy Mimiaga:** 51 (both) **Dan Mooney:** 50 **National Park Service:** 26, 62, 65, 83 (both) **Pikes Peak Cog Railway:** 154, 156 (bottom), 157 (both) **Shine and Deesa Rogers:** 6, 23 (bottom), 174, 178 (both), 179 **Shutterstock:** 23 (top) **Gordon Slabaugh:** 42, 43, 44 (both), 46, 47 **The Seven Falls Company:** 184, 185 **Norm Thompson/courtesy of Glenwood Caverns Adventure Park:** 100 (both) **Sandy Tradlener:** 50 **Ute Mountain Tribal Park:** 200 (top), 201 **Ellen Wadley:** 45 (both)

Artwork credits by artist and page number:
**Julie Martinez**: 9, 12,14, 17, 18 **Vernon Morris**: 31, 64, 93, 110, 119, 127, 128, 131, 144, 153, 161

Cover and book design by Jonathan Norberg

10  9  8  7  6  5  4  3  2

Copyright 2007 by Jon Kramer, Julie Martinez and Vernon Morris
Published by Adventure Publications, Inc.
820 Cleveland Street South
Cambridge, MN 55008
1-800-678-7006
www.adventurepublications.net
All rights reserved
Printed in China
ISBN-13: 978-1-59193-208-6
ISBN-10: 1-59193-208-4

## Special Thanks

Sometimes we spend months on end living the glorious adventurer's lifestyle. Oh sure, there's the quiet spirituality of waking at sunrise, tucked away in a remote red canyon with ancient cliff ruins all around. And then we have those incredible Kodachrome sunsets you can only experience from crystalline mountain peaks. But, just as often, it's a hard, gritty, elemental existence, altogether sweaty and clammy, testing your resolve and sometimes your sanity: One day you're hunkering down in a desert sandstorm that's incessantly blasting your sorry butt into rawhide, the next you're getting frostbitten fingers and freezing your gonads in a mountain peak snowstorm. It's at times like these when you might say to yourself, *What am I doing in this torture pit? I wish I had a friend or relative living near here, so I could escape this God-forsaken hole! Oh, for a hot shower, warm meal, clean bed . . .* Lucky for me I have just exactly that sort of escape hatch in Colorado. My Aunt Priscilla—a wonderful charmer and provider—has fed and sheltered us all countless times on our Rocky Mountain adventures. We are grateful to her and her late husband Dave for enriching and preserving our lives.

Strange and humorous as it may sound, I have to give a long-overdue special thanks to my *Cocci*-brother George who, during our geology field camp in Florissant several years ago, showed true friendship above and beyond the call of duty by picking cactus spines out of my butt after I cleverly embedded them there while sitting on a hidden barrel cactus. I highly recommend you do not try "cactus riding" yourself as it is unlikely you will have such a dedicated friend as George nearby in your moment of agonizing need.

On a recent blustery October morning I found myself on an impromptu visit to "Eldo" (climbing lingo for Eldorado Canyon) lamenting the fact I didn't have my climbing gear. Not surprisingly I stumbled upon fellow climbers—Matt and Clayton Conrad—snaking up routes along Wind Tower (see listing for Eldorado Canyon). I stopped and talked story for awhile, carefully lacing my dialog with subtle hints such as, "It's a tricky layback on that flake up there. If I had my gear I'd show you a few moves . . . " Once they realized I wasn't a "poser," they tossed me a harness and the short end of the rope. A few climbs later and I was stoked for the rest of the week. Thanks for the tune-up guys.

Special thanks are deserved by many who've opened their doors and hearts to us along the way despite the fact we sometimes smelled bad, maybe ate too much food, probably drank all the beer, and very possibly ruined the washing machine. Among these nobles are: Joe Dallas Glenn, of Mt Princeton Hot Springs. Erin Lee at Royal Gorge. Fred Oglesby of Rio Grande County Museum in Del Norte. David Donatto at Pikes Peak Cog Railway. The kids and teachers of Douglas County.

# TABLE OF CONTENTS

## Welcome to Colorado

What is it about mountains that make them so compelling? Is it their size, their snowy tops, their airy heights? Is it the different environs they harbor on their flanks, the dichotomy of lush green base to icy cold summit? Or is it something ethereal inside each of us that prompts a longing to be among them? Colorado has some of the most beautiful mountains in the lower 48 states and that's just one reason to go.

But there's a lot more to Colorado than mountains. There are canyons as deep as the Grand Canyon, sand dunes as high as the Empire State building, and ancient ruins tucked away in hidden alcoves high on cliff walls. There are monster huge dinosaurs and delicate fossil butterflies, bellowing elk and busy hummingbirds. There are hot springs, cold springs and warm springs.

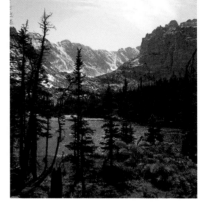

Colorado is a land of endless diversity and great natural beauty. We could write reams but it'd just scratch the surface of all the great places here. So, we're going to get real and just list our favorite sites, keeping things as mixed up and diverse as possible. Our entries are brief summations designed to give you a realistic feel for what's here. They are intended as a tool for you to plan your own adventure, be it by foot, mule, bicycle, car, RV, or your own private space ship.

We do not restrict our listings here to government-sponsored sites or strict non-profit organizations. To be sure, some of the best natural wonders in Colorado are on private property, not reliant on tax dollars or grants for support.

We've enjoyed the splendor of Colorado's ancient, rugged natural beauty. We've been traipsing around the state for decades—trudging up mountains and down canyons (and sometimes the other-way-around), hiking through deserts and riparian areas, swimming in the cooling pools of a hidden waterfall—all in pursuit of the truest nature of the state.

We hope you have as much fun as we've had exploring the mountains, valleys, canyons and mesas of Colorado. It's a journey of adventure.

Keep in touch!

Jon, Julie, & Vern

## Keep In Touch

In 1896 an Irish immigrant carpenter, Thomas Walsh, bartered for, and acquired title to, an abandoned mining claim near Ouray, Colorado. He got it for a song, primarily because the land had no gold. The former owners had dug themselves silly but never recovered a thimbleful of the lustrous yellow metal. Yet Thomas was no fool, he'd been staying up late at night to teach himself everything there was to know about geology and the precious mineral. He bought the mine knowing full well he wouldn't find any gold. But what he did find bothered him.

Thomas found what he thought looked like telluride—an ore of gold—all over the place. It had been blasted out of the mountain and discarded by the former owners while sinking their shafts in pursuit of native gold. But there was so much of it lying around it couldn't possibly be gold telluride—it had to be something else. There was no way the seasoned miners before him would not have recognized such a mineral for what it was. Or maybe . . .

The Luck of the Irish must have followed Thomas over from the Emerald Isle because when the assay came back, he realized his ship had come in. A big ship, in a big way! The Camp Bird mine ultimately became one of the richest gold strikes ever and Thomas Walsh quickly became one of the wealthiest men in the world. A few years later he bought the Hope Diamond for his daughter, with little consideration to the price.

So what does all this have to do with our little guidebook here and the title of this section? Well, nothing. I just thought it was a pretty cool story to pass on about Colorado. But there is a footnote: Whenever Thomas Walsh was away, which was quite often, he always wrote back home about his adventures. These became cherished reading for his daughter Evalyn who eventually published a book about her dad called *Father Struck It Rich.* In the book she continually praised her father for his letters. So the moral of the story is to keep in touch—write us a line or two about how you've enjoyed these sites. And if you have any sites of your own which belong in a book like this, we're happy to check them out. If we use them in the next edition, you'll receive full credit and a gift from us personally. Just don't count on getting a gold mine cheap!

Contact us at: www.JourneyGuides.com

or, write us at:

Colorado Journey Guide
c/o Adventure Publications, Inc.
820 Cleveland Street South
Cambridge, MN 55008

# Using This Guide

## About the listings

When you glance at this map the first thing you think is—"What's with the site numbers scattered all over the place?" Now slow-up a little, there's a reason: All the sites are in alphabetical order by name. So, naturally, they do not follow any sort of geography. Every site we list— be it on private, public, or reservation land—is open to the public as of the date of this printing. But things change and it's always good to confirm by phone.

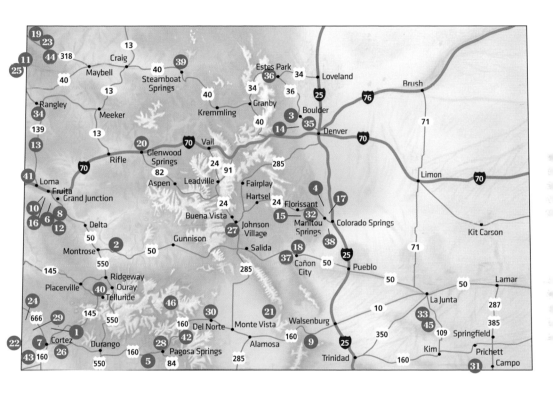

## Ratings

In the Rating of each entry we give you an idea of the quality of experience you can expect with that aspect of the site. Our ratings are, admittedly, subjective. You may not agree with what we think all the time but you'll get the hang of it. The ratings are determined by our own personal standards. For the record, we take into account the quality and quantity of the subject matter, its educational value and presentation, and our overall impression of the experience visiting the site. We use a scale of 1–5 stars with some plus or minus for in-betweens. Like in the hotel trade, five stars is top honors. Here's an approximation of how we rate things:

★☆☆☆☆   B-O-R-I-N-G and/or barely worthy of note, but for some reason we listed it anyway. Don't waste your time by going out of the way to see this one.

★★☆☆☆   Stop by here if you're in the area and need to kill time. Who knows, you may like it more than the rating suggests.

★★★☆☆   Definitely worth a visit, no excuse necessary. Even if it means going a little off course to see it.

★★★★☆   This place warrants a detour and/or change of plans to visit although you might want to stop short of divorcing your partner to get here.

★★★★★   Shazzam! This site is worthy of quitting your job and hitchhiking cross-country just to catch a glimpse of it. Go ahead, divorce your spouse if you need to—it's worth it!

After the ratings for each site, you'll note the category in parenthesis. This means that the site is rated in one or more of the following areas:

> archaeology
>
> geology
>
> paleontology
>
> museums

Therefore, the following entry would mean that this site is archaeologically significant, in Jon's opinion, but only mildly significant geologically.

**Jon's Rating:** ★★★★☆ (archaeology)

★☆☆☆☆ (geology)

★★★★☆ (museum)

# Access

The ease with which you can access the main aspects of each location is indicated by a generalized rating of its own. **Do not take this as gospel!** Remember, you are responsible for your own well-being. Things change all the time, especially in the no-man's land of some of these places. Check beforehand with local land managers if you have any question about the difficulty. (And by the way, we've included the contact information so you can't complain to us about not knowing who to call for a road and trail condition report.) In some cases, we indicate the difficulty of access by car to the trail head versus the difficulty of the trail itself. Trail rating is loosely defined along these lines:

### Easy
No real problem. The site is nearby parking or within a short, easy walk. If there are any complaints you've taken the wrong path.

### Moderate
Usually requires some hiking over moderate topographic relief. No need for swearing and little-to-no sweat.

### Difficult
Prolonged and/or rough hiking over significant topographic relief. There's likely to be some sweating here and the trek may occasionally warrant foul language.

### Extreme
Very difficult, often multi-day hiking among rugged, remote terrain. Use of foul language and inappropriate gestures probable. Requires profuse sweating under arduous circumstances. Use deodorant.

Many places have multiple sites, some easy to access and others downright extreme. Such places will have a range of ratings that apply. For instance, Mesa Verde has an Access rating of Easy–Difficult. A car or bus tour of the top is easy. If, however, you wish to hike in places such as the Pictograph Trail, then you're in for more of a challenge.

# Introducing Colorado

## Archaeology

 Some of the most famous archaeology in the world is in the mesas, mountains and canyons of Colorado. What we have here, as they say, is a fairly comprehensive listing of all the publicly-accessible archaeology sites in the state at the time of printing. We don't, however, attempt to document every single site you might be able to visit had you 3 weeks, Ironman endurance, a tanker-load of water, and a dedicated chuck wagon. After all, the vast majority of Colorado archaeology sites have yet to be documented and many of these are on public land. But we do list those which a normal everyday traveler can access in one day with reasonable effort in decent weather.

We will not attempt to educate you on all the ins and outs of the various waves of human influence, occupation, and cultures which play a role in the natural history of Colorado. Suffice to say, the list is long and very diverse. The archaeology here, as in most places, is in a constant state of revision, with new sites and new theories being discovered almost weekly. But researchers generally agree on the basic major Pre-Columbian cultural influences in Colorado and those are shown in the table to the right.

**Note on discovering new sites:** If you happen to come across what you think may be a new archaeology site, please do not disturb anything. Take photos, note the exact location on your map or GPS, and notify the office of the State Archaeologist. Your reward is knowing you did the right thing. Also, consider this added bonus: by virtue of doing nothing at such a site you avoid jail time and bad publicity. Archaeology sites—including rock art—are very strictly protected by law.

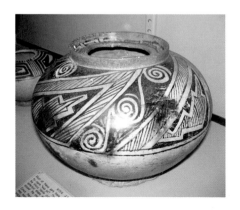

# APPROXIMATE CHRONOLOGY OF PRE-COLUMBIAN CULTURES IN COLORADO
### (using revised Pecos classification)

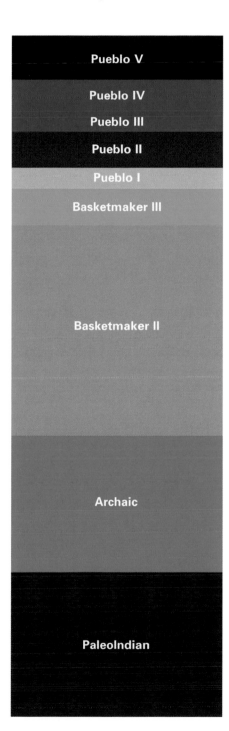

| | |
|---|---|
| Pueblo V | 2000 |
| | 1900 |
| | 1800 |
| | 1700 |
| | 1600 |
| Pueblo IV | 1500 |
| | 1400 |
| Pueblo III | 1300 |
| | 1200 |
| | 1100 |
| Pueblo II | 1000 |
| | 900 |
| Pueblo I | 800 |
| | 700 |
| Basketmaker III | 600 |
| | 500 |
| | 400 |
| | 300 |
| | 200 |
| | 100 AD |
| | 0 |
| | 100 BC |
| Basketmaker II | 200 |
| | 300 |
| | 400 |
| | 500 |
| | 600 |
| | 700 |
| | 800 |
| | 900 |
| | 1000 |
| | 2000 |
| | 3000 |
| Archaic | 4000 |
| | 5000 |
| | 6000 |
| | 7000 |
| | 8000 |
| PaleoIndian | 9000 |
| | 10,000 |
| | 11,000 |

Cultures in the Colorado area

Cultures in all of North America

# Paleontology

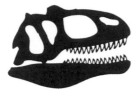

Colorado is rich with fossils, many of which are on public land. Paleontology sites on all public lands (whether local, state, or federal) are protected by laws, although the exact details and applications thereof are yet being refined by the authorities. Unfortunately, most bureaucrats don't know a fossil from a turnip and this causes confusion and inconsistency in land-regulating policy. Still, ambiguity in the law does not allow you license to collect fossils willy-nilly.

Understandably, the rules governing fossil collecting on public land are designed to keep the activity under control and to aid in the promotion of the science. All one has to do is look at the devastation in some areas, such as some fossil fish sites in southern Wyoming, to see the wholesale destruction wrought by unregulated collecting and basic human greed. There are some fossil collecting sites which look more like a cratered moonscape than a scientific excavation.

So before you run off to dig merrily for fossils on BLM land, you need to understand a few things. First off, learn the difference between a vertebrate, invertebrate, and plant. (We're not gonna re-teach you this—you should remember it from elementary school biology. If you don't, ask your kids or go to the library.) The second part is easy. Essentially the rules for collecting fossils on U.S. public land go something like this: Vertebrates–NO, Invertebrates and Plants–YES, with some restrictions.

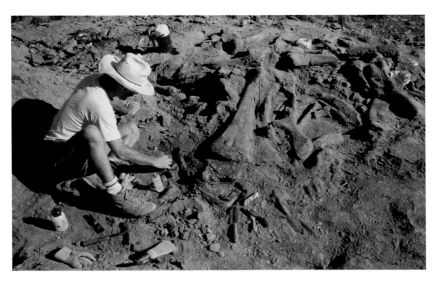

**Vertebrates:** You personally cannot collect any fossils of vertebrate animals on U.S. public land without a permit. Period. That means you won't be running out and chasing down dinosaurs on your own. But if you're dead set on digging dinos or other vertebrates, there are options—you can team up with any number of professionals that run field camps in the summer months. Check local clubs, universities and museums for these opportunities. It's hard, tedious, work, but very rewarding.

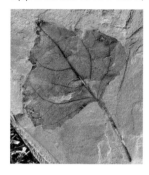

**Invertebrates and Plants:** There is some good news for the intrepid fossil collector in you and it concerns fossils of invertebrates and plants, which are, happily, far more abundant than vertebrates. According to the BLM, which publishes a handy little brochure on fossil collecting called Fossils on America's Public Lands (circular number: BLM/WO/GI-97/006+3032+REV06), "You may collect a variety of invertebrate and plant fossils on BLM public lands, with certain restrictions." The fossils you collect in this manner must be for your own enjoyment and cannot be bartered or sold. In addition, some particular areas may be off limits to all fossil collecting (such as Dinosaur Hill, Fruita Paleo Area), and others may have more refined rules. Check with the local BLM office ahead of time for the real scoop on fossil collecting in a given area.

State and local public lands have their own rules for fossil collecting and you must find out from the local land managers what's what in these areas before you search for fossils on them. Private land is another matter altogether. The law is clear here: Fossils on private land belong to the land owner. You may dig to your paleontological heart's content on private land so long as you have a contract and/or permission from the owner.

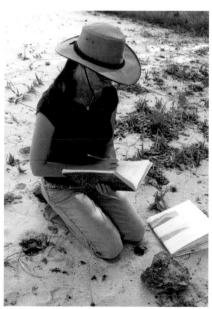

**Keep notes:** Regardless of what you find, keep notes with the specimen as to where exactly it was unearthed, the date, and any particulars that may be of interest to researchers. A specimen becomes scientifically worthless without this information. Half the fun of finding a fossil is learning more about it and you start by keeping notes.

**Paleo organizations:** If you have an interest in fossil collecting we strongly encourage you to join a club. The largest and most active in Colorado is the Western Interior Paleontology Society (WIPS website www.wipsppc.com) which holds monthly meetings at the Denver

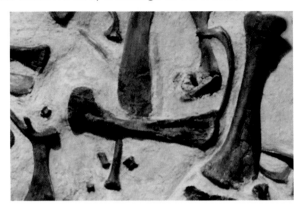

Museum of Nature and Science. If you become truly serious about paleontology we further recommend that you consider going through the Denver Museum of Nature and Science Paleontology Certification Program (see their website at www.dmns.org). This program not only teaches you techniques of paleo field and lab work, but can also be an entree into other opportunities in the science. At the very least you should ally yourself with an institution and a professional paleontologist in your area. They can help you in learning about your discoveries. In exchange, you may be able to help them with their research. You might even get a new species named after you! It's a win-win situation when we all work together to advance the science.

# Geology

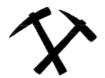

Colorado has a long geologic history and an important fossil record. The oldest rocks in the state are Precambrian granites which form the "basement" of the Rockies, while the youngest are Pleistocene and Holocene sediments scattered as thin crusts atop older rocks in river valleys and creek beds.

Colorado is further blessed with a great diversity of geologic provinces, landforms, and outcrops. Nearly everywhere you look in this state there are unique and exciting geologic features, from the towering peaks of Rocky Mountain National Park to the deep fissures of Black Canyon of the Gunnison. Because a large portion of the state is public land, you're welcome to explore many of the wonders of this geologic cornucopia. But let's face it, even in a dozen volumes, there wouldn't be enough room to describe all the great geology here. So we're gonna take the easy way out and only discuss the highlights which are fairly accessible to you. Keep in mind all the archaeology and paleontology sites have some sort of geologic aspect to them, so even if you don't see mention of them in the listing, you'll doubtless enjoy the added geo-bonus free of charge.

| | Years (millions) |
|---|---|
| **CENOZOIC ERA** | |
| Holocene Epoch | |
| Pleistocene Epoch | |
| | 2 |
| **Pliocene Epoch** | |
| | 5 |
| **Miocene Epoch** | |
| | 24 |
| **Oligocene Epoch** | |
| | 35 |
| **Eocene Epoch** | |
| | 55 |
| **Paleocene Epoch** | |
| **MESOZOIC ERA** | **65** |
| **Cretaceous Period** | |
| | 140 |
| **Jurassic Period** | |
| | 200 |
| **Triassic Period** | |
| **PALEOZOIC ERA** | **240** |
| **Permian Period** | |
| | 290 |
| **Carboniferous Period** | |
| | 360 |
| **Devonian Period** | |
| | 410 |
| **Silurian Period** | |
| | 440 |
| **Ordovician Period** | |
| | 500 |
| **Cambrian Period** | |
| **PRECAMBRIAN** | **570** |
| **Proterozoic Eon** | |
| | 2500 |
| **Archean Eon** | |
| | 3600 |
| **Pre-Archean Eon** | |
| | 4500 |

## Visitor Etiquette

### Irreplaceable Treasures

We're quite sure you don't need to be told that the sites you'll visit are fragile, irreplaceable, natural treasures. We're also certain you don't want to hear again and again that these sites need your care in preserving them. And, really, why would we want to use valuable print space to tell you how important it is for you to take an interest in conserving these sites for future generations when we all know you understand and practice that already? What with all those laws and societal taboos in place to ward off destructive behavior, who in their right mind would even consider such negligence? Certainly not you or us. But you never know. You may come across someone who doesn't understand these things—say a social deviant, cultural moron, or an alleged human with the collective intelligence of a brick. If you do, you can just show them this paragraph and try to set them on the straight and narrow path. God smiles on those who help preserve the Earth.

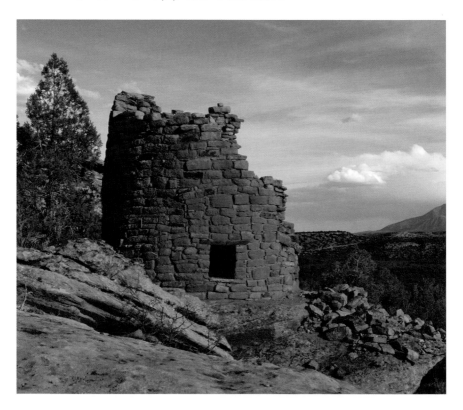

## Do Not Disturb

Let's suppose you stumble across a huge pile of broken pottery or a petrified log weathered into thousands of fragments at a place not mentioned in this or any other guidebook. You might reason that pocketing just one tiny piece or two couldn't possibly impact the site as a whole, considering the uncountable abundance still left undisturbed, right? No, not right. In fact, VERY not right. If every visitor took just one tiny piece then soon there would be nothing left except an empty hole where once there was a dinosaur skeleton or a cliff dwelling. So please don't do it, don't disturb any sites. Future generations will thank you. And you'll be doing your part in relieving over-crowded prisons by not becoming an inmate.

## Precautions

### Snowstorms

Remember this: Mountains can rearrange your priorities in a hurry.

In the summer of 1976 I went west with some high school buddies. We spent time visiting friends in Pagosa Springs at the base of the San Juan mountains. The climber inside got the best of me so I ditched my friends for a day and headed out to a couple of 14ers over near Ouray.

It was late June and I was looking forward to a good little workout with a day-long, alpine-style, speed ascent up one or both of the peaks I was cycing. The previous few days had been sunny and warm—nearing 80 degrees in the valley.

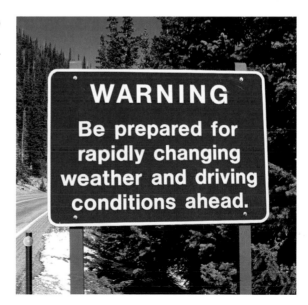

In true alpinist style, I went with only the barest minimum of gear—a water bottle, a wind breaker, and a couple candy bars. When I left the car it was a nice sunny day.

But then it got windy. Then it got cold. Long before I got within sight of any summit, I was freezing my butt off. I thought "What the hell, I know what I'm doing here. I climb mountains, I can make it. It's not like this puny mountain is gonna kill me or anything . . ." Then the storm hit—the wind was howling and the snow (yes snow!) was thick, washing in tidal waves over the ground. The wind chill must have been zero or below, and it was classic "white-out" conditions. Very deadly.

In severe white-outs you cannot—dare not—move. If you do, you're guaranteed to lose your way, and quite possibly your life in the process. All you can do is hunker down and ride it out. I spent my time crouched beside a boulder, cursing the situation and my own colossal stupidity. I should have brought some warm clothes! What a fool I was.

If the storm had lasted, I wouldn't be here to tell you about it. When the snow finally abated, I was so cold I could hardly walk! But I dragged my sorry butt off that blasted rock pile as fast as I could go. Needless to say the summit was no longer a priority. Suddenly, just staying alive was a major battle. I got out with no real injury, except to my pride—it was the first summit I didn't make—but pride takes a back seat to survival. I'm happy to report there have been many "unmade" summits since that day, a fact that only bolsters my confidence. Since then I've learned what my limits are—what to bring and when to retreat. As a result, I get a lot of mileage talking about my "unmade summits." After all, there's little to say if you die in an attempt. Mountaineering is all about coming back alive.

The moral to the story is, in the mountains you have to be aware that weather can change in a hurry. One minute it can be sunny and warm, the next it can be sleeting or worse. Exposure to cold is a very real threat every week of the year. Do not underestimate the possibility of hypothermia, global warming notwithstanding. People die of exposure every year in the mountains, many in mid-summer.

## Bring Lots of Water

Colorado is both hot AND cold, depending on where you go and when. Many of the 14ers have snow pack on them in July and August and we all know about the famous snowfall in the mountains during the winter. During the summer, the lowlands and canyons become stratigraphic ovens that can fry a rock. So be prepared for hot or cold climate anytime.

Bring plenty of drinking water wherever or whenever you go, even in winter. Many of these sites are remote and have no water supply.

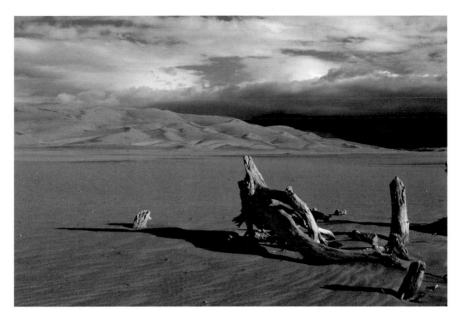

Here's a lesson in common sense: just because a site is named something provocative like "Big Bozo Spring" doesn't mean there's a spring there. Or, if there is, it may be undrinkable (such is the case with most of the 150 springs in the Steamboat Springs area). Also, we've jumped on to the Better Health Bandwagon and are promoting a reduction in skin cancer, so stock up on sunscreen and wear a wide-brim hat. Sunscreen and sun glasses are imperative anytime in the mountains.

If you're camping in the desert, be aware that it can get chilly at night, even in the summer. In the winter, the higher elevations and plateaus can become veritable deep freezes with temps down below zero not uncommon. And don't forget the wind! The wind can become a major force to be reckoned with, especially if it's cold. As they say in Minnesota—"Bring warm clothes!"

## Rock Fall

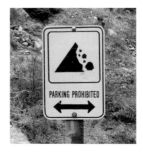

Remember that story in 2003 about Aron Ralston the explorer who was climbing through a Utah canyon when a loose boulder shifted and pinned him against the wall? He was trapped for days before he finally did the unthinkable and cut off his own arm with a pocket knife so he could escape. He made it out alive, but just barely.

In the wilds, the dynamics of weathering ensure a continual supply of loose rock and precariously balanced boulders, especially in the mountains. We recommend you do not tempt fate by scrambling around off established routes. If you do take the path less traveled be sure to hike with a companion. We want you to come home with all your limbs intact and with stories a little less harrowing than Aron's. Keep in mind that steep mountainous terrain can be host to major rock slides, especially during spring thaws.

## Flash Floods

Do not enter any canyon, creek, river, or wash if there is a chance of rain in the region. Read that last sentence again and pick up on the word "region"—meaning not just the immediate area, but any place within the watershed of your area. This is especially important in narrow canyons during spring runoff or in major thunderstorms.

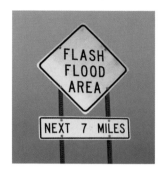

## Roads

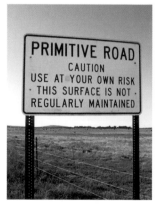

A great many of the sites we list are accessible by pavement and/or maintained gravel roads. Many others are attained via unimproved dirt tracts that can be dicey in bad weather, even for 4WD. We strongly recommend you check locally about road conditions before heading out to remote sites. If you don't, you may be in for a long hike back out and enormous tow-truck charges. Most of these sites do not need 4WD but be sure to use caution anywhere the road is unmaintained.

## Animals

Most of the time you'll not encounter bothersome animals. Pay attention to some simple rules of thumb and you're not likely to have a problem with them:

- Never, EVER!, feed the wildlife. You've heard it before but we'll tell you again: Feeding wildlife encourages dependency on unnatural food sources and may lead to unwanted advances—advances which may not end when you want them to.

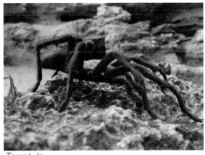
*Tarantula*

- Don't approach wild animals—observe and record them from a distance.

- Live with compassion—enjoy, but do not harass, other living things. This a good principle applicable to animals as well as plants. It should be observed by people as well as governments. Although it's often ignored by the latter, we hope you, at least, take the message to heart. Even the tarantulas of Mesa Verde (they love ruins too!) are an important part of the environment, so please drive around them when you see one on the road (they like warm pavement on cold mornings).

No matter where you go or when, we strongly recommend you research the area you are traveling to in order to become familiar with the wildlife you'll encounter. Here is a short list of animals which you should be aware of in Colorado: Mountain lions, coyotes, bobcats, and

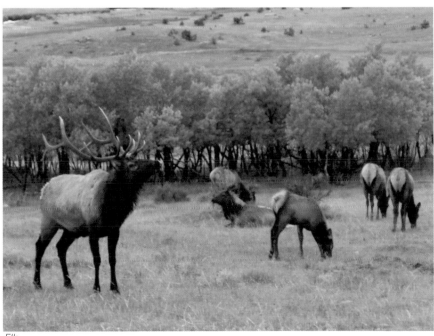
*Elk*

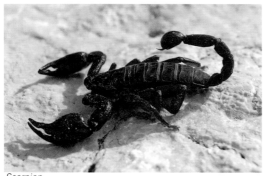
*Scorpion*

Javalinas are just a few of the mid-size mammals that can, if necessary, inflict real pain on humans. Just follow the rules above and you're likely to avoid this. Bears don't care much for people and you can avoid them by keeping your camp clean and food stored properly in your vehicle or bear locker. Elk and moose are obviously huge mammals that can plow you down with little or no reason—don't give them one. Even deer can be lethal—in Yosemite National Park, for example, deer are the only animals responsible for human deaths in recent years. Also, in the summer months, certain other critters come out to play: Scorpions, tarantulas, rattlesnakes, Gila Monsters, and bees are potentially harmful to humans. Remember, you are just a visitor in their world, so tread softly. Keep an eye out—don't put your hands or feet where you cannot see them, especially under rocks or in crevasses. With a little common sense we can all get along.

## Plants

Plants of the desert are another matter altogether. Cactus are ubiquitous throughout much of the state's lowlands and even in the high parks. Be careful where you tread. DO NOT sit on the ground without first checking the spot or you may find yourself asking a travel partner for some unsavory help. This is EXACTLY what happened to me in South Park several years ago when I plopped down onto a well-camouflaged barrel cactus. You learn

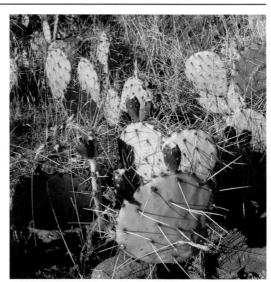
*Prickly pears welcome you to the desert.*

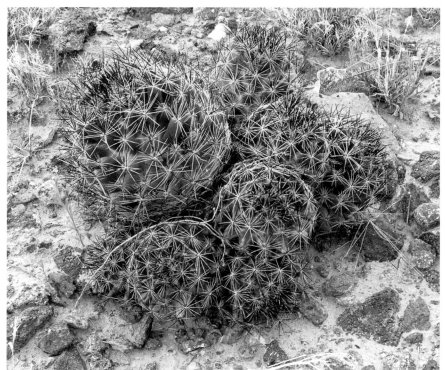
*Cactus can be a painful experience.*

what friendship really is when you ask someone to excavate cactus spines off your sorry ass. Believe me, it ain't pretty—from any angle. (Thanks again, George!) Maintain a bit of distance from cactus and you'll be fine.

## The Best of Colorado

If you had to choose just one site from each category that was the absolute top of its class, which would it be? The following are our choices for the best of the best of Colorado:

### Archaeology

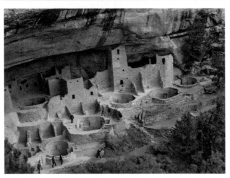

There are many very excellent archaeological sites in Colorado. The problem is picking one place which best represents the diversity and quality of the archaeological experience. The runner-up spot in the competition has to be Ute Tribal Park, host to an archaeological experience unlike any others. But the winner, not surprisingly, is **Mesa Verde National Park**, the place that has it all: cliff dwellings, petroglyphs, pictographs, caves, ruins of all kinds and everything in idyllic canyon settings that are very easy to visit.

### Paleontology

Colorado is famous for its fossil record. There are many superb pre-historic specimens—from dinosaurs to mammoths—which have been unearthed here. If the Dinosaur Quarry of Dinosaur National Monument was actually in the state, we'd say this was a good contender for the best of Colorado as far as paleontology is concerned. But it's not, so that's that. Stop your crying.

Call me biased (I had a geology field camp here in the 80s), but I have to elect **Florissant Fossil Beds National Monument** as the premier

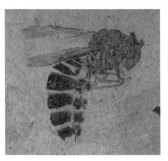

fossil location in the state. The fine "paper shales" of Florissant make for remarkable fossil preservation—unlike any other. Delicate butterflies look like they were flying around here just yesterday. Leaves seem as though they just fell from the trees. Fossils of fish and insects show remarkable details. The sheer variety as well as quality of the fossils is unsurpassed by any other site in North America. The only deficit is the lack of a decent visitor center or museum. For decades the park has struggled to obtain funds for a proper overhaul of the tiny facility it now hosts. But the lack of visitation and its out-of-the-way location has worked against it. Although the present facility is small and in need of updating, the outdoor displays of fossil sequoia stumps are mind-blowing. The beauty of the fossils and the setting they are in are unsurpassed. And here's an added bonus: you can dig your own fossils just outside the park at the small private quarry there.

## Geology

Here again there are some close contenders for the title "Best of" title. Certainly we must include Rocky Mountain and Great Sand Dunes National Parks. But the rule is we have to pick just one to be the Best of Colorado Geology, so **Black Canyon of the Gunnison National Park** is it. In our opinion it holds the most amazing geology you'll see in one place in Colorado. It's deep, it's narrow, and it's beautiful. Unlike the lazy soft-rock lithology of the Grand Canyon in Arizona which is rather predictable from one end to the other, Black Canyon is made up of primarily hard-rock metamorphic

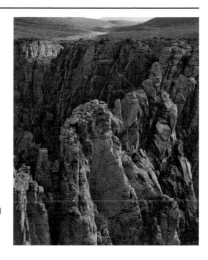

Black Canyon Gneiss that cannot be "sorted out" easily. Wild, chaotic intrusions of pink pegmatites spider-web throughout its sheer walls, producing such splendors of nature as the Painted Wall. Although megalithic displays of metamorphosis are not uncommon throughout the world, Black Canyon is certainly among the best.

## Museums

On page 210, we've listed the notable museums related to Archaeology, Paleontology, and Geology. Keep in mind we do not attempt to list all museums (e.g., the Old West Museum or the Doll Museum) as spell-binding as they may be, simply because they are not applicable to the type of journey you are reading about here.

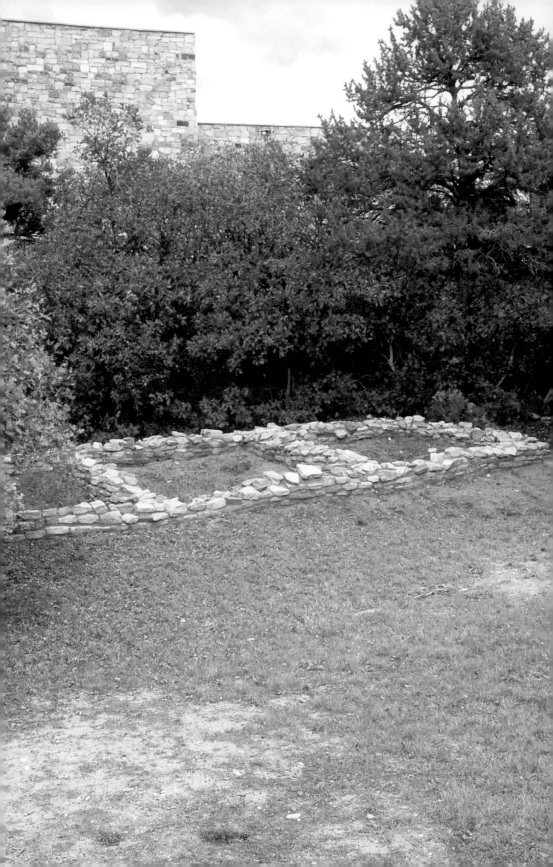

# ANASAZI HERITAGE CENTER

## I

**Directions:** From Cortez head north on CO 145 about 9 miles. At the intersection with CO 184, head west, away from Dolores. About a mile or so down the road you'll see the Anasazi Heritage Center which is the main visitor center for the monument.

**Contact Info:**
Anasazi Heritage Center
970-882-4811
www.co.blm.gov/ahc/hmepge.htm

**Fee:** no fee to see the ruins; museum at heritage center has a modest entrance fee and it's worth it!

**Hours:** park open year-round; heritage center hours 9am–5pm March–Oct, 9am–4pm Nov–Feb; closed on Thanksgiving, Christmas and New Year's Day

**Best time to visit:** anytime, but the heat of mid-summer can roast you; if you go in July or August make it as early in the day as possible, otherwise go in the off-season to avoid the crowds and heat; I like October the best

**Camping/Lodging:** basic camping on BLM land for free, but not in, or next to, any ruins. Nearest lodging in Cortez.

**Access:** easy, paved trails at the center, replete with ranger-led programs

**Jon's Rating:** ★★★★★ (archaeology)

**Jon's Notes:**
Apparently there were a lot of "Ancients" as well as a lot of Canyons here, so the BLM maxed-out the creativity meter and came up with a very ingenious title for this monument: *Canyons of the Ancients* (as opposed to say, "Steep Valleys of Some Long-Ago Folks"). Despite the name, the monument itself is incredible and this particular local-ity operates as its very exciting visitor center. Not only is this an education complex but it's also a full-blown museum which curates over three million artifacts from southwestern Colorado. There's even a few real pueblos on-site to make you feel at home.

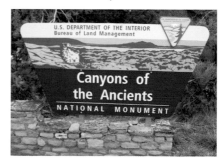

*LEFT: A fine museum surrounded by ancient ruins.*

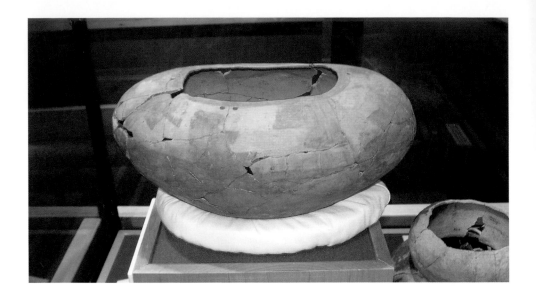

The museum houses
reconstructions of
ancient dwellings
as well as artifacts
excavated from the
nearby ruins.
The diversity and
abundance of the
ceramics alone is
amazing.

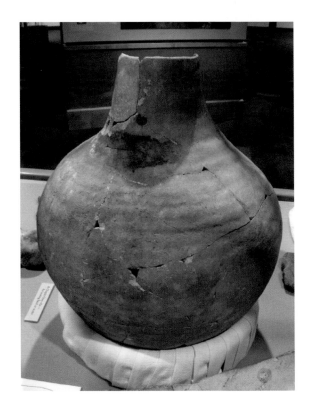

## CANYONS OF THE ANCIENTS

It's doesn't have the giant, gazillion-room cliff dwellings of Mesa Verde or Ute Mountain Tribal Park, but neither is it crowded like those places. In fact there's a good chance you won't see anyone at all in the outer areas and that'll enhance your experience by leaps and bounds. Canyons of the Ancients effectively encompasses everything else left over after the Utes got their reservation and Mesa Verde got its park. The ruins are prolific, unspoiled, and, for the most part, unexcavated. Do your part when visiting the ruins by observing the rules and minimizing your impact. (Artwork by Vernon Morris)

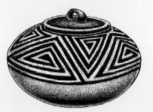

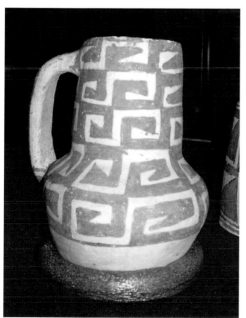

*Anasazi beer stein or Aunt Jemima syrup pitcher? Probably neither, but it sure would work for lemonade.*

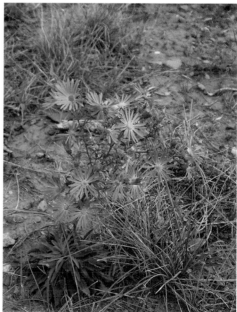

*Native wild aster.*

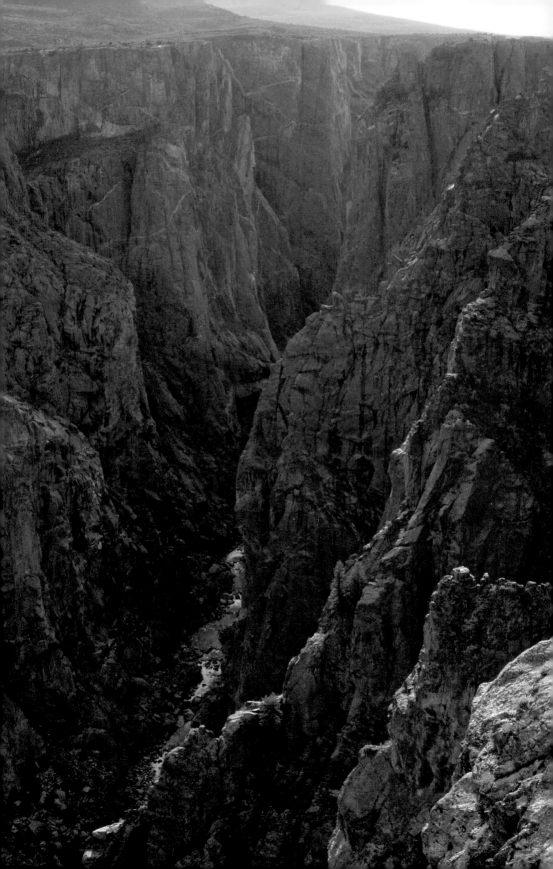

# BLACK CANYON OF THE GUNNISON NATIONAL PARK

**Directions:** From Montrose follow US 50 east 8 miles to CO 347. Head north 5 miles to entrance.

**Contact Info:**
Black Canyon of the Gunnison NP
970-641-2337
www.nps.gov/blca

**Fee:** vehicle entrance fee

**Hours:** park open year-round; visitor center hours are seasonal

**Best time to visit:** summertime is the most crowded but also the nicest weather; since the rim is at a higher elevation, the temps are usually moderate even in mid-summer; I recommend September—the crowds are gone and the weather is still enjoyable

**Camping/Lodging:** improved camping in the park spring–fall; camps closed in winter; nearest lodging in Montrose

**Access:** hiking along the rim is easy; anything else—like going down to the river—can be everything from moderate to extreme

**Jon's Rating:** ★★★★☆ (geology)

**Jon's Notes:**
Colorado is a land of kinetic geology. Its vast mid-section is an evolving mountainscape, while the north and south have dynamic landforms of their own—mesas, plateaus, buttes, and canyons. It should come as no surprise to anyone that some of these features go beyond just your everyday, garden-variety "wow." One of Colorado's truly magnificent places is the canyon formed by the Gunnison River. Not only is it good and deep, but the thing which really puts this one in the "awesome" arena is the fact you can easily see the other side, a vision which defies description. Contrast that with the Grand Canyon of Arizona fame where all you see is endless canyon upon canyon, upon canyon. At times it's just too much of a good thing.

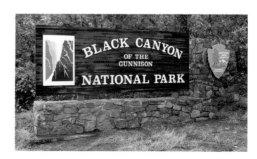

*LEFT: The chasm . . .*

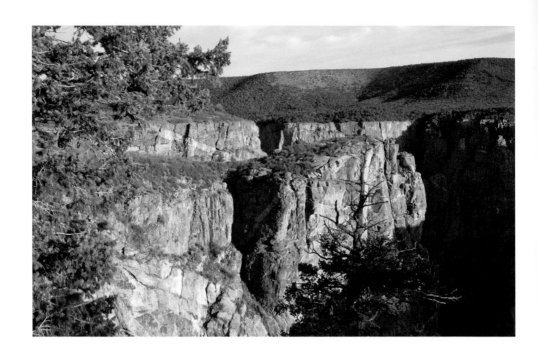

*It's a jumble of metamorphic rock and it gets pretty deep. The nice thing about this place is you can see across to the other side from most points along the rim.*

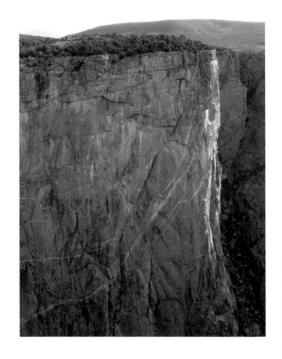

## META ZIGZAGS

Unlike that other Grand Canyon to the southwest which is composed of layer upon layer of boring sandstone and limestone, this one has a much more impressive lithologic repertoire. The Gunnison River has been plowing its way through metamorphic rock that's both harder and more wild in its twisted, mashed appearance. The wild scatters of lighter-colored zigzags apparent in the huge walls are mostly pegmatite dykes of various size and structure. They intruded into the massive metamorphic rock long after it had cooled and hardened. Along came the Gunnison, carving its way through the amalgam and giving you something worth your praise.

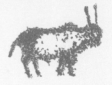

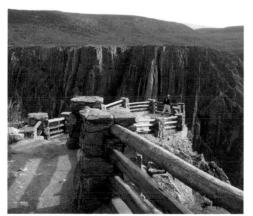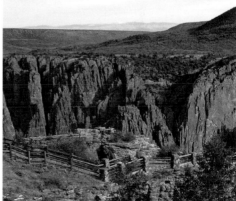

*The Visitor Center is, not surprisingly, situated at one of the best overlook areas to view the dynamic geology of this incredible chasm. But, worry not, the paths at this particular spot are all well-protected.*

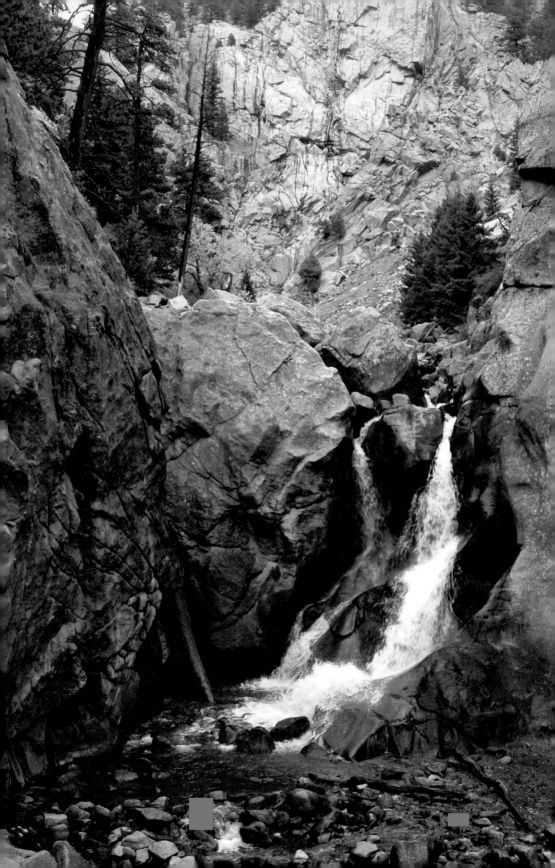

**Directions:** Boulder Canyon is along CO 119 west of Boulder. The falls are about 10 miles out of town, while the best part of the walkway is about half that far, marked by signage on the left.

**Contact Info:**
City of Boulder
303-441-3440
www.bouldercolorado.gov/index.php?option=com_content&task=view&id=2875&Itemid=1016#Boulder%20Falls

**Fee:** no fee

**Hours:** daylight hours

**Best time to visit:** anytime the road and trail are not too icy

**Camping/Lodging:** camping nearby; closest lodging in Boulder

**Access:** easy—but be careful near the falls—the rocks can be very slippery

**Jon's Rating:** ★★★☆☆ (geology)

**Jon's Notes:**
There are falls all over this state and a lot that are many times higher than this. So why do we list this one? Stop off to see it and you might actually learn a lesson or two about geologic processes. Never has such a fall been so appropriately named. In this case it's not just the fact it occurs on the north branch of Boulder Creek, but that there is actually a gigantic—and I do mean GIGANTIC!—boulder that is the star of the show. The huge litho-leviathan dislodged from the wall of the canyon above and somehow managed to become wedged in the V-shaped narrows downstream, effectively blocking the flow. Afterward, a small lake built up behind the pinch and eventually the water coursed over the top, a process which continues today.

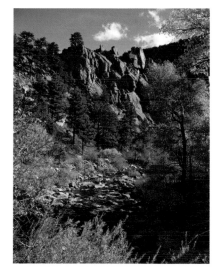

*LEFT: A rolling stone gathers no moss. But a giant boulder that gets stopped dead by wedging itself in a mountain stream might very well gather some moss, as well as a lot of water behind it.*

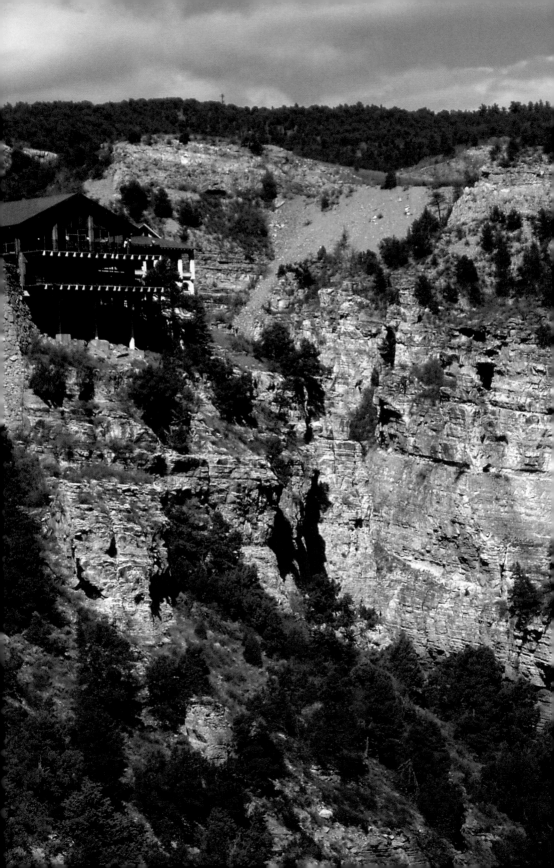

# CAVE OF THE WINDS

## 4

**Directions:** The cave entrance is located just outside Manitou Springs, off US 24. Look for the hole in the ground, or just follow the signs.

**Contact Info:**
Cave of the Winds
719-685-5444
www.caveofthewinds.com

**Fee:** per person entrance fee

**Hours:** summer 9am–9pm; winter 10am–5pm

**Best time to visit:** anytime

**Camping/Lodging:** camping and lodging in Manitou Springs and Colorado Springs

**Access:** easy underground hike on mostly paved trails, though you may feel a little claustrophobic at times

**Jon's Rating:** ★★★★☆ (geology)

**Jon's Notes:**
There's only a couple of caves in Colorado which are open to the public and this is one. It's not Mammoth Cave of Kentucky nor Kartchner Caverns in Arizona, but it is one of the more realistic caving experiences you'll encounter. The long and winding passages are narrow—most were never widened since their original discovery—and the low ceilings in some parts make you feel right at home as a troglodyte underground.

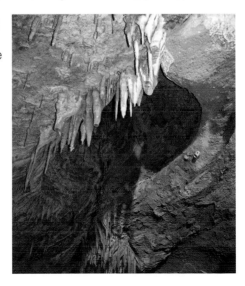

*LEFT: On a picturesque cliff above Manitou Springs is one of Colorado's easiest caving adventures.*

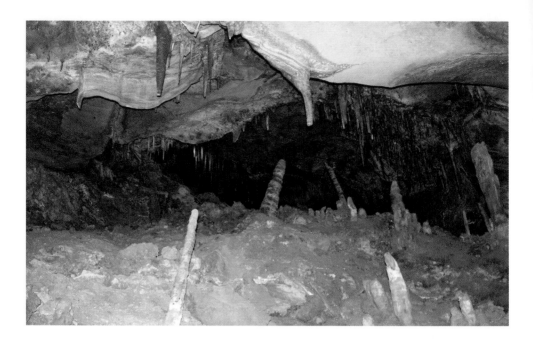

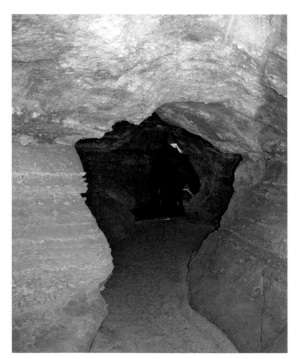

*There's something pretty cool about wandering around underground.*

*ABOVE: Stalactites and stalagmites abide in many places along the tour.*

*RIGHT: The tour follows natural passageways.*

## LET'S HAVE SOME RESPECT

Cave conservation is all the rage these days and the science of speleology has finally entered the commercial cavern industry, albeit a bit late. Back in the day, cave patrons were encouraged to maximize their underground experience by taking home a piece of the rock, as it were, and more than a few did just that. In the early days of most commercial caverns, the overeager over-did it and the result was a great denuding of the insides. Cave of the Winds is no exception—countless stumps of broken-off stalactites and stalagmites lie along the pathways and the once-impressive soda straw grottos have been reduced to a shadow of their former glory. However, some of the most important formations—from a strictly speleological standpoint—are the helectites. They are both numerous and well-protected.

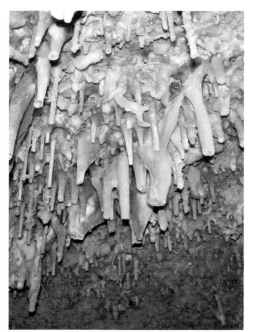
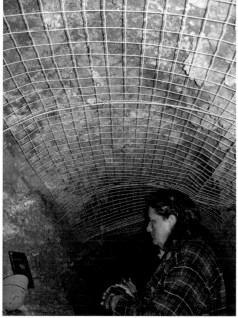

*Cave of the Winds is doing its part in cave conservation by not allowing you to touch the formations. In areas that are close to the paths, barriers (right) protect the formations (left).*

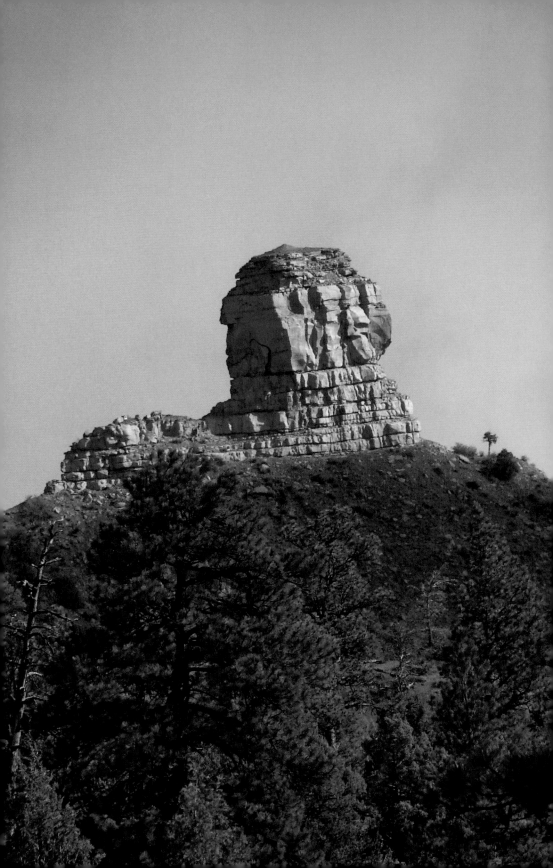

# CHIMNEY ROCK ARCHAEOLOGICAL AREA

## 5

**Directions:** From Pagosa Springs follow US 160 west 17 miles to CO 151. The visitor center is about 3 miles south.

**Contact Info:**
Chimney Rock Visitor Cabin
970-883-5359
www.chimneyrockco.org/

**Fee:** per person entrance fee

**Hours:** May 15–Sept 30, daily 9am–4:30pm

**Best time to visit:** anytime in the summer; the site is closed in the winter but it does host special events; check the website

**Camping/Lodging:** camping at Ute Campground nearby; nearest lodging in Pagosa Springs

**Access:** moderate hike around the mesa top

**Jon's Rating:** ★★★★☆ (archaeology)

**Jon's Notes:**
The Chimney Rock complex is composed of eight clusters of residential structures that cover a time range of 850–1125 A.D. during the Ancestral Puebloan cultural development periods. The prehistoric inhabitants of Chimney Rock first entered the North Piedra River valley area as farmers. By 950 A.D. the people were moving to the high mesa tops where they utilized reservoirs and diversion ditches to farm and provide drinking water. Chimney Rock eventually attracted the attention of the major Ancestral Puebloan center at Chaco Canyon, 93 miles to the southwest. It is believed that Chimney Rock became part of the larger Chacoan regional community as an outlier or satellite community.

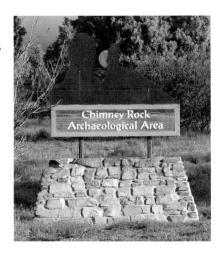

*LEFT: It sort of looks like a chimney . . .*

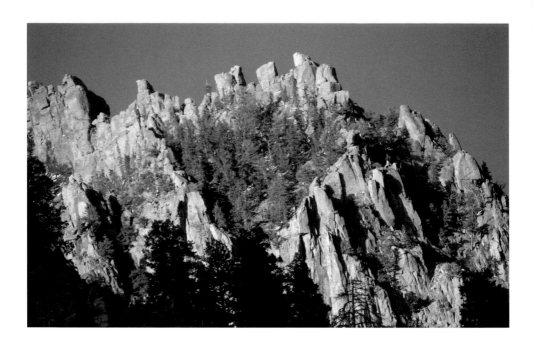

*There's a whole lot of geology going on here but that's only half the story. The primary precipitous pinnacle—Chimney Rock (right)—was so compelling to ancient people that they built a pueblo nearby.*

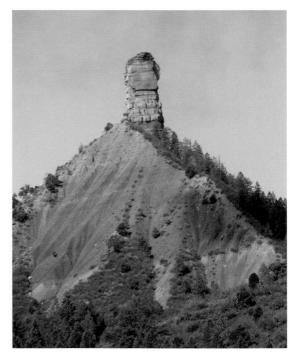

## YOU CAN HAVE YOUR CAKE AND EAT IT TOO!

Used to be you had to decide between studying the stars or ancient civilizations. But now, in the modern Age of Multidisciplinarianism, if you have a knack for ancient cultures and astronomy you're in luck. A fairly new scientific field affords you the luxury of doing both—it's called archaeoastronomy. You may already know that certain ancient monuments and ceremonial structures were astronomically aligned. Stonehenge in England and the Great Pyramids in Egypt are outstanding examples. But did you know we have some home-grown archaeo-astronomy sites of our own right here in the hood? In 1988 a rather interesting celestial phenomenon was observed at Chimney Rock by an enterprising professor. Dr. J. McKim "Kim" Malville, from the University of Colorado, theorized that the Ancestral Puebloans probably used Chimney Rock's pinnacles in the observation of astronomical events called "lunar standstills." He has also observed similar events at Mesa Verde and Chaco Canyon, evidence which suggests these cultures were far more sophisticated than originally thought.

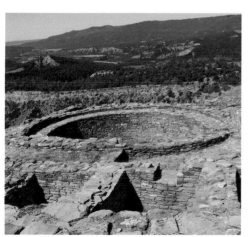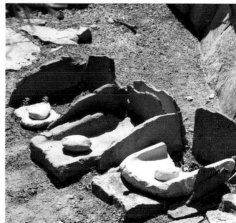

*Researchers surmise that Chimney Rock may have been an important archaeoastronomy site. Excavations continue to yield clues.*

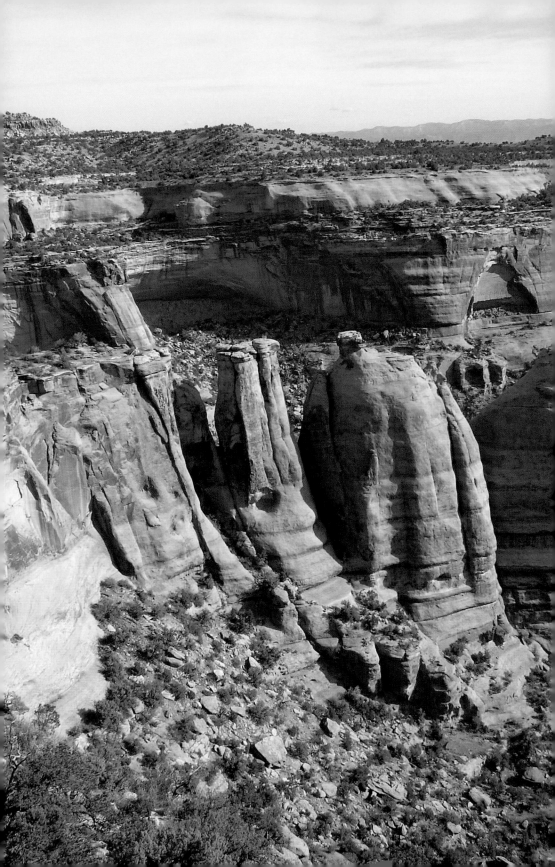

# COLORADO NATIONAL MONUMENT

## 6

**Directions:** From Fruita, follow CO 340 southeast 4 miles to Rim Rock Road then follow the signs to the monument visitor center.

**Contact Info:**
Colorado National Monument
970-858-3617
www.nps.gov/colm

**Fee:** vehicle entrance fee

**Hours:** summer 8am–6pm, winter 9am–5pm

**Best time to visit:** anytime the weather is good and even most times when it's not; people get married here all the time!

**Camping/Lodging:** improved camping in the monument campground; lodging in Fruita

**Access:** easy–difficult; the drive is, of course, easy but well worth it; hiking can be whatever you want up to extreme

**Jon's Rating:** ★★★☆☆ (geology)

**Jon's Notes:**
You might think a place in Colorado that's named Colorado National Monument is a bit presumptuous. But remember there also happens to be a river by that name and that's what this name refers to. The Colorado flows right through this monument and has carved some mighty impressive canyons, buttes, and mesas along its course. The emphasis is on geology here, with a myriad of formations exposed and glowing along the canyon lands. It's a good primer for trips to the Grand Canyon or Bryce and Zion, but is a lot less hassle than any of them.

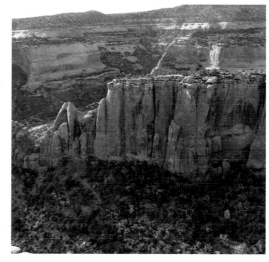

*LEFT: It's a great place to hike or drive. It's not a bad place to get married either.*

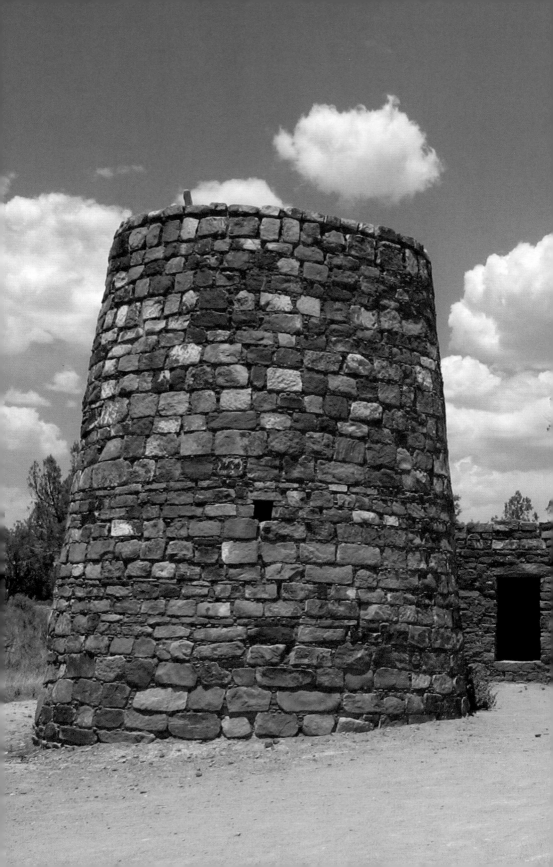

# CROW CANYON ARCHAEOLOGICAL CENTER

**Directions:** From Cortez, follow Hwy 491 north about 1½ miles, staying in left lane. Watch for Crow Canyon sign on the right side of the highway. Turn left (west) on Road L. Drive about 1 mile (watch for Crow Canyon sign). Turn left onto Road 23. In about 1 mile, Road 23 curves to the left and turns into Road K, which in turn becomes Crow Canyon's driveway.

**Contact Info:**
Crow Canyon Archaeological Center
800.422.8975
www.crowcanyon.org/index.html

**Fee:** fees are based on type of program

**Hours:** day tours offered twice a week in the summer; field camps and research weeks are ongoing; check the website

**Best time to visit:** anytime they have tours

**Camping/Lodging:** improved camping and lodging in Cortez; summer camps have lodging on campus

**Access:** easy

**Jon's Rating:** ★★★★½ (archaeology)

**Jon's Notes:**
You are not likely to encounter an institution quite like Crow Canyon Archaeological Center anywhere else. This 170 acre "campus" is not only home to impressive collections of ancestral Puebloan artifacts from around the region, but it also includes accurate recreations of pit houses and pueblos. In addition, the Center is a hub for field and laboratory research in the entire Mesa Verde region, publishing scientific research on a regular basis. The best news for you is it's open to anyone with a semi-serious interest in archaeology. You can dive in for a little or a lot.

*LEFT: The Center has several full scale "ruins" reconstructed on the property.*

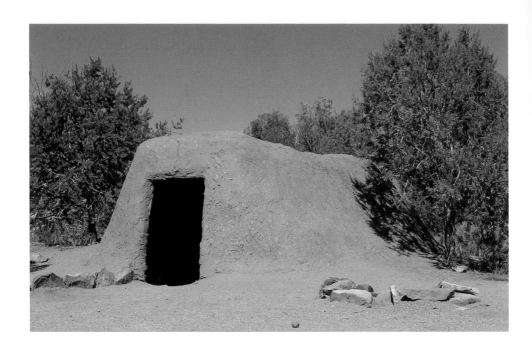

*There's no better way to get a feel for how ancient people existed than to build some of the structures they lived in.*

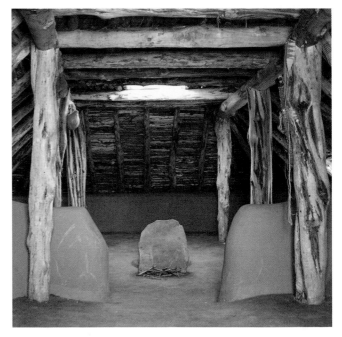

## BACK TO SCHOOL

Crow Canyon Archaeological Center is one of the most ambitious and distinguished campus-based educational complexes in the world of archaeology. The hands-on programs allow you to participate in actual archaeological research, making exciting discoveries in the field and laboratory that add to our understanding of the Puebloan past. The Center's research and education programs are developed in consultation with American Indians, whose insights complement the archaeological perspective and add a unique cross-cultural dimension to your experience.

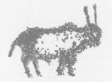

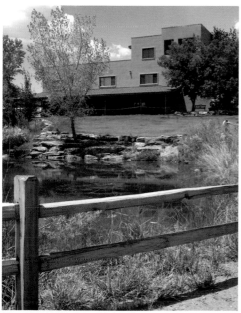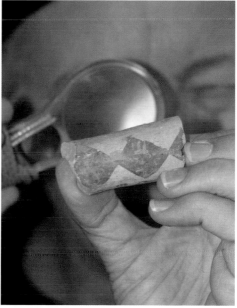

*The campus also houses full research facilities complete with conservation labs where researchers can study the collections.*

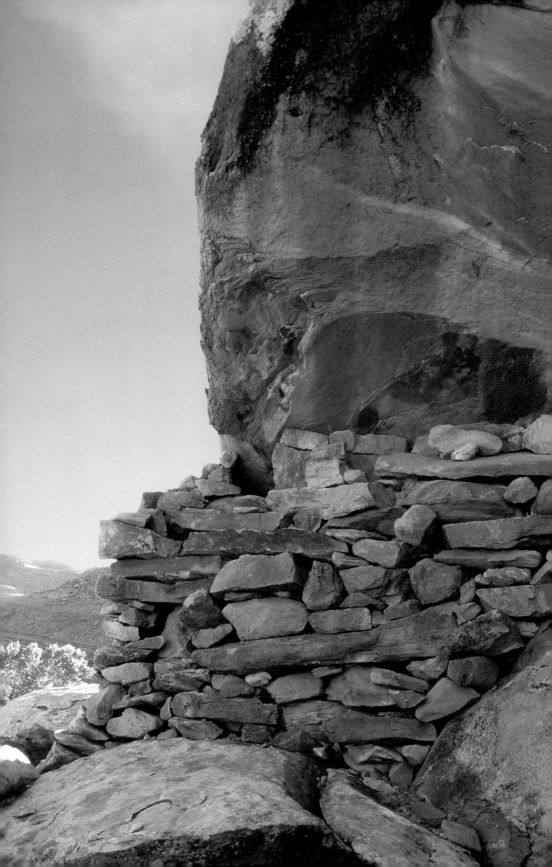

# DEER CREEK PETROGLYPHS

## 8

**Directions:** From Grand Junction follow US 50 about 20 miles south-east to mile marker 52. Turn west onto Bridgeport Rd. and follow 3 miles to the parking area at Gunnison River. It's a very short hike from the parking area at the river. The petroglyphs abide on the largest boulder at the base of the mesa corner formed by Deer Creek and Gunnison River, just north of the parking area. **You cannot see the rock art from the parking lot**, so look for the biggest boulder north of the road and head to it. You will cross the creek immediately off the road and in 5 minutes be at the site.

**Contact Info:**
BLM Grand Junction Field Office
970-244-3000
www.co.blm.gov/gjra/gjra.html

**Fee:** no fee

**Hours:** year-round daylight hours

**Best time to visit:** whenever the weather is good

**Camping/Lodging:** basic camping on BLM land; nearest lodging is in Grand Junction

**Access:** easy hike to the boulder at the base of the mesa where the site is

**Jon's Rating:** ★★✦★★ (archaeology)

**Jon's Notes:**
Below the giant boulder lies a small structure built by who-knows-who way-back-when. The large panel of clear petroglyphs runs adjacent to the area of the structure along the west-facing surface of said boulder. Neither the structure nor petroglyphs are visible from the road, being blocked from view by a slightly smaller group of boulders. So you'll have to get to the site to see it. But the trek is easy and fairly short. Other sites are in the area (see Dominguez Canyon) across the river but are much more remote and if I told you how to get to them, they'd have to kill me.

*LEFT: Nothing like a gigantic boulder to anchor your home-sweet-home against.*

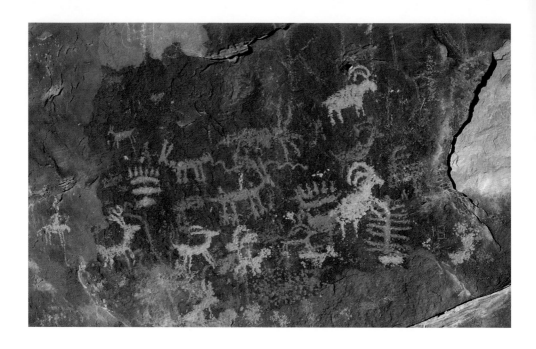

Hey, when you love art, hanging it outside your house isn't such a bad idea. Petroglyphs of animals and abstracts cover the boulder surface just outside the structure.

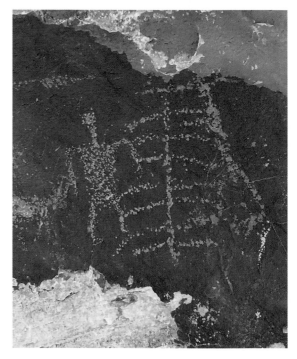

## HEY! IS THAT REALLY A BASALT BOULDER THERE?

Along the road to see the petroglyphs you will notice a very official BLM sign declaring "Bridgeport Basalt Boulder Site." Hurray! Someone recognized the obvious—there are basalt rocks here, some of which might even classify as boulders. Ignoring the fact that basalt is ubiquitous over the entire region, the question becomes what exactly is the big deal here? We stopped and investigated the spot twice and both times we came away stymied, not knowing even if the sign referred to a geologic, archaeologic, historic or some other type of "site." Are there hidden petroglyphs on the boulder surfaces? We never found any. Could the ancients have aligned the rocks for shelters or made geoglyphs or sleeping circles? If so, it certainly isn't evident now. Or perhaps it's a geologic site—maybe the boulders here contain some rare lithologic character. Whatever it is, there's no info at the "site." We concluded the sign probably refers to space alien abductions. It does seem there are less and less of the rocks every time we go by the place, and we all know how those space aliens like basalt boulders . . .

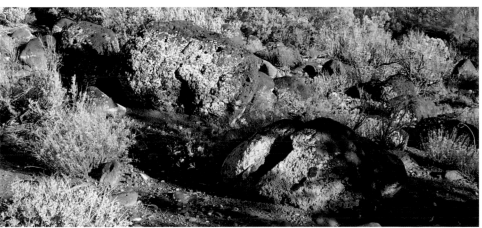

*Yep, they're basalt all right!*

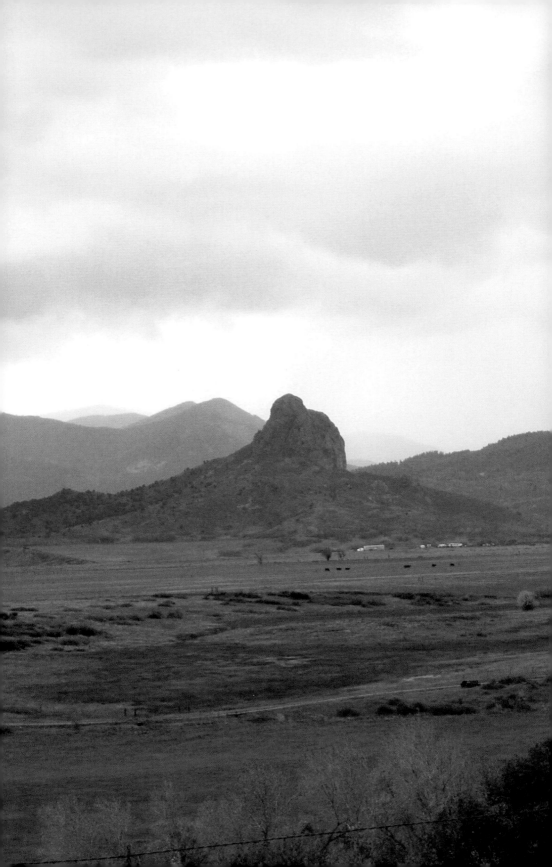

# DEVILS STAIRSTEPS

## 9

**Directions:** From Walsenburg travel west on US 160 for 11 miles, then south on CO 12 through the town of La Veta. About 7 miles south of town look for mile marker 11.5 and the signage at the base of the "steps." Hopefully, the devil will have left by then.

**Contact Info:**
No visitor center—no phone
www.spanishpeakscolorado.com/Devils.html

**Fee:** no fee

**Hours:** year-round daylight hours

**Best time to visit:** when the sky is blue!

**Camping/Lodging:** camping and lodging in La Veta

**Access:** easy, since you end up staying in your car, there's not much in the way of hiking here

**Jon's Rating:** ★★⯪☆☆ (geology)

**Jon's Notes:**
It's been awhile (like maybe 5 million years, but who's counting . . . ) since things were booming in the tiny town of La Veta, but that doesn't slow them down any. This idyllic and progressive little town south of US 160 is home to artists, ranchers, entrepreneurs, and more than one excellent cook. In addition to hosting famous street fairs the town also happens to be situated among some textbook examples of structural geology. West of town is the prominent volcanic neck of Goemmer Butte, once a conduit for magma heading to the surface.

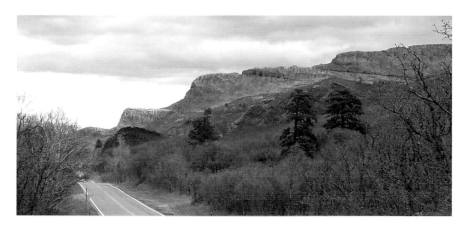

*LEFT: The place is covered with volcanoes. The throat of one just outside town.*

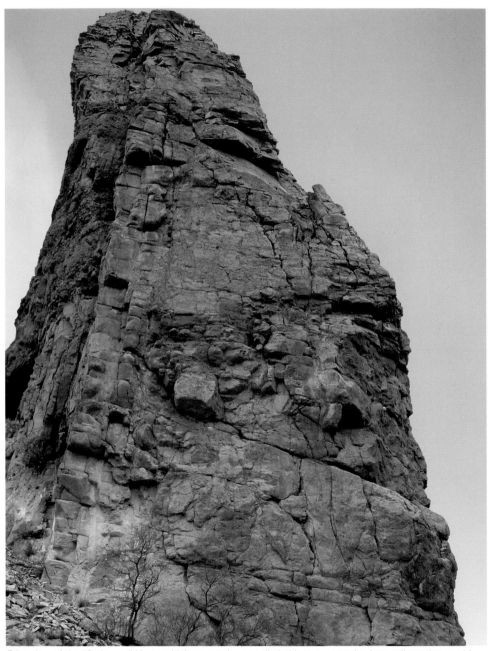

*Edge-view of the "Staircase." You wouldn't want to have to climb this to get upstairs, I can tell you that much!*

## FAULTY DIKES

South of town are the real geologic treats—uncountable numbers of radial dikes spreading from the Spanish Peaks like a spider web of fractured glass. The Devils Stairsteps are a result of weathering along the brow of some of these dikes. These features are a product of the Spanish Peaks "intruding" into the older rocks of the area and forcing their way to the surface. Faulting is prolific in such a scenario with dikes forming along such lines of instability. But here the dikes are especially abundant and easily-identified. Add to that the good news there's evidence faulting is still going on in the area, and we're likely to see geology classes making field trips here indefinitely.

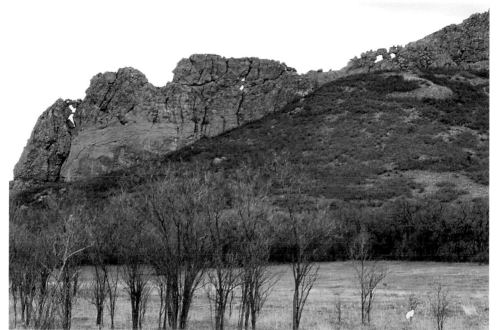

*The devil is gonna have to do some maintenance on these if he expects to keep using them. These steps are rotting to pieces!*

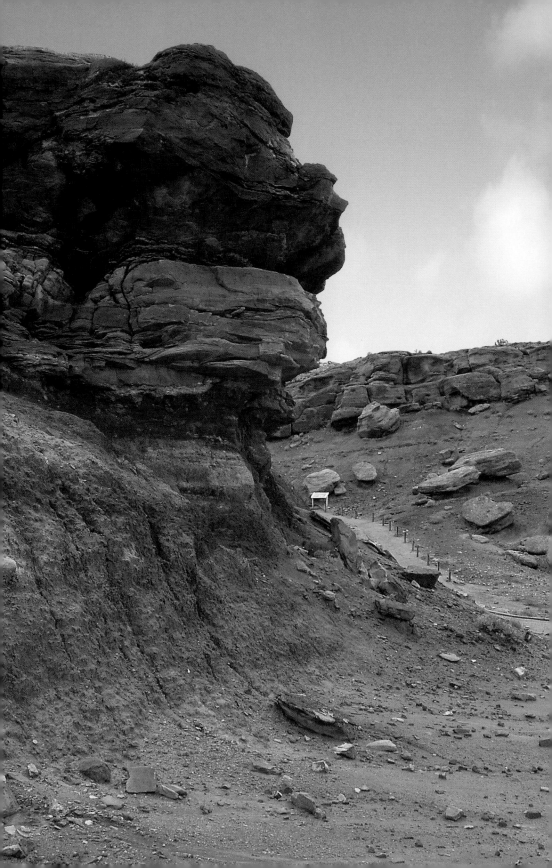

# DINOSAUR HILL

## 10

**Directions:** From I-70 in Fruita, go south on CO 340 about 1 1/5 miles to the signs for the parking lot. There is a hill, dinosaurs notwithstanding.

**Contact Info:**
BLM Colorado
970-244-3000
dinosaurdiamond.org
www.co.blm.gov/mcnca
www.dinosaurjourney.org

**Fee:** no fee

**Hours:** year-round daylight hours

**Best time to visit:** when the weather is good; not much fun in the rain or snow

**Camping/Lodging:** improved camping and lodging in Fruita and Grand Junction

**Access:** easy access and easy hike around the hill

**Jon's Rating:** ★★☆★★ (paleontology)

**Jon's Notes:**
At one time there were live dinosaurs at Dinosaur Hill. At one time there were dead dinosaurs at Dinosaur Hill. But now there are no dinosaurs at Dinosaur Hill. Sorry, but that's the way it is at Dinosaur Hill. It's a sad fact you'll discover once you've tramped around the small butte in search of the elusive giant bones. BLM and local groups have, however, done their best to preserve the history here. Like Graceland minus Elvis, they've cranked up the wow-o-meter by selling the sizzle. Graphic-rich signs and maps tell you why this place has a claim to fame but, as they say, Elvis has left the building.

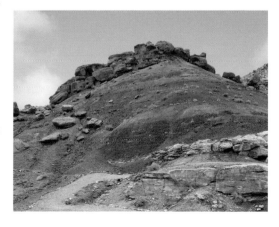

*LEFT: Yes, there's a hill, but the dinosaurs got away . . .*

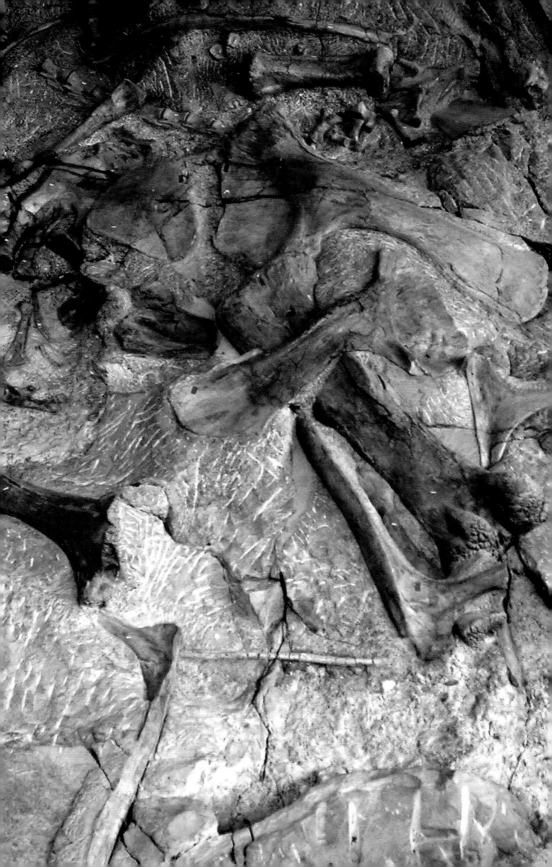

# DINOSAUR NATIONAL MONUMENT

## II

**Directions:** The monument straddles both Colorado and Utah. The best petroglyphs and the only dinosaur bones on display are on the Utah side. Go there! From Jensen, UT travel north on UT 149 about 6 miles to the visitor center and bone quarry.

**Contact Info:**
Dinosaur National Monument
970-374-3000
www.nps.gov/dino

**Fee:** vehicle entrance fee

**Hours:** park open year-round; visitor center hours are seasonal

**Best time to visit:** Whenever they reopen the quarry! Barring that, it's nicest in the fall.

**Camping/Lodging:** improved camping in the monument, lodging in Vernal or Dinosaur

**Access:** easy–moderate; driving is easy—most of the roads are paved and there are lots of great sites along the road; hiking the back country can get pretty difficult especially on a hot summer day

**Jon's Rating:** ★★★½★ (geology)
★★★★★ (archaeology)
★★★★½ (paleontology)

**Jon's Notes:**
"Quarry closed!" was the greeting I got after a long drive from the Black Hills. I checked the calendar—no, it wasn't a holiday, so what's with the sign? As my luck would have it, the Dinosaur Quarry—which houses the only visible dinosaur bones in the entire park—was closed for an indefinite period of time. It seems the structure built overtop of the bone bed was deemed unsafe just the day before. The rangers were all apologetic but had no idea when this wholly untenable situation would be remedied. "Hopefully within a year," was one's guess. Hopefully? Considering governmental slo-mo and bureaucratic bungling, you better check before planning to see the famous bones for which this place is named.

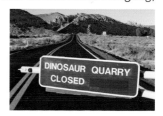

*LEFT: You'll go completely ga-ga when you see the bones in the quarry. IF you even get a chance to see the bones in the quarry.*

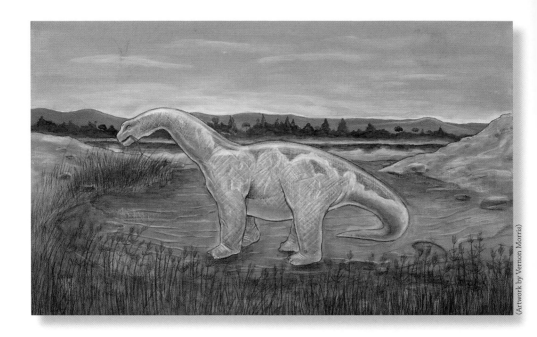

(Artwork by Vernon Morris)

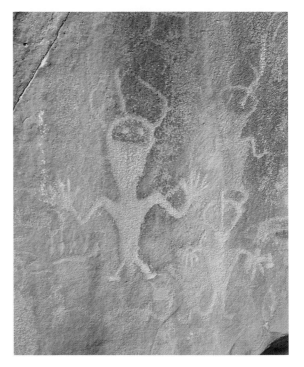

Even if the quarry isn't open, that's no reason to pass up this jewel of a National Monument. As the brochure says, there's so much more to Dinosaur than dinosaurs. If the geology doesn't completely fill your adventure cup, check out the archaeology—sites abound inside the park boundaries and many are nearby the roads.

ABOVE: Many of the skeletons in the dinosaur quarry are from Camarasaurus.

RIGHT: The great rock art of Swelter Shelter.

## SWELTER SHELTER

Not far down the road from the bone quarry—toward the campground— is a small but impressive rock alcove. Named Swelter Shelter by the 1966 crew who excavated it in searing heat, this important site has yielded hundreds of artifacts—spear points, scrapers, hammer stones and others. One of the greatest attributes is the shelter's unique rock art—an uncommon combination of petroglyphs and pictographs found together in the same image. These gems of prehistory were scribed in at least two phases by Freemont artists about 800 years ago. The subtle art is yet clearly visible today.

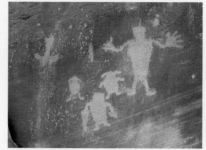

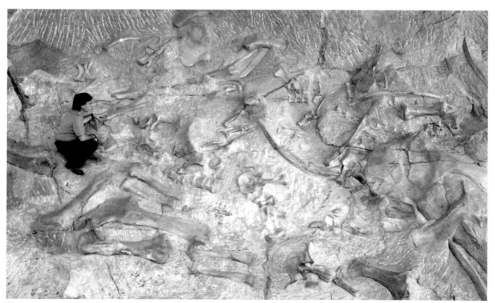

*Here you can dig dinos without digging them. But that's only if the dinosaur quarry reopens before you go.*

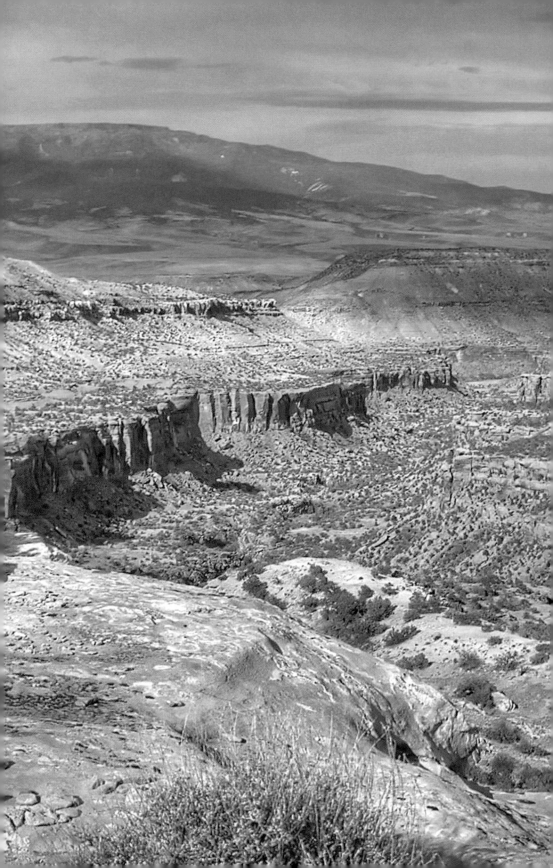

# DOMINGUEZ CANYON WILDERNESS STUDY AREA

## 12

**Directions:** From Grand Junction follow US 50 about 20 miles southeast to mile marker 52. Turn west onto Bridgeport Rd. and follow 3 miles to the parking area at Gunnison River. The footbridge is 1 mile upriver from the parking area and another mile up the Gunnison River the trail turns and enters Dominguez Canyon. Half a mile up the canyon is the confluence of Big and Little Dominguez Creeks and a mile or so upstream from the confluence you will find several large boulders with petroglyphs right on the hiking trail.

**Contact Info:**
BLM Grand Junction Field Office
970-244-3000
www.co.blm.gov/gjra/dominguezwsa.htm

**Fee:** no fee

**Hours:** year-round daylight hours, best time between May and October

**Best time to visit:** avoid mid-summer heat or mid-winter snows; I like fall or spring the best

**Camping/Lodging:** basic camping on BLM land in the Dominguez Canyon Wilderness Study Area. Nearest lodging is in Grand Junction

**Access:** moderate 3.5 mile hike (one-way) to the petroglyphs, but the canyon itself is beautiful and the hike very scenic

**Jon's Rating:** ★★★★☆ (geology)
★★★☆☆ (archaeology)

**Jon's Notes:**
If you find yourself checking out the Deer Creek site, you'll notice the driving directions are essentially the same here. The difference is you must hike about 3½ miles one-way to see the petroglyphs while the Deer Creek site is right near your car. But the scenery is worth every step, especially once you get into the canyon. We advise you camp a night or two here—it's fantastic. Be sure to bring plenty of water.

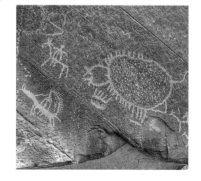

*LEFT: It's not Bryce or Zion, but it's a lot easier to get to.*

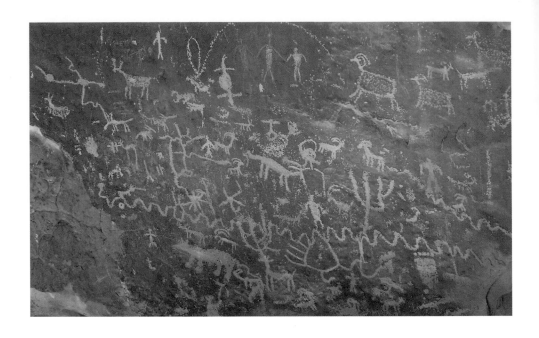

The trail can be long on a hot summer day, but it's always scenic and there are great petroglyphs right beside it.

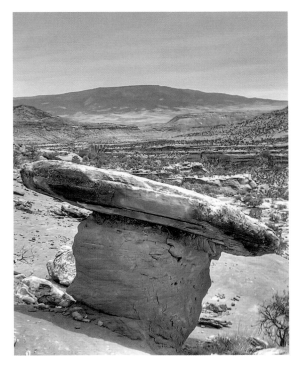

## WILDERNESS AREAS

On the surface of it, designating certain places as "wilderness" may seem like a bureaucratic maneuver designed to cash in on pork-barrel politics. Once you visit them it's not really necessary for someone to remind you of the fact that the place is wilderness to the core. There's often little in the way of improvements—the whole idea of wilderness is a lack of such things. And, the best part is you're not likely to encounter Paris Hilton or Rush Limbaugh schlepping a pack through remote canyons of such places. However, as redundant as it may seem, wilderness areas do require special consideration because of their fragile nature. The BLM and Park Service have adopted a special idiom in such areas called **Leave No Trace**. It's a good policy wherever you travel but is especially important in wilderness areas. The idea is exactly what it says—please try to leave no trace of your passing through such areas. Visit www.LNT.org to learn more.

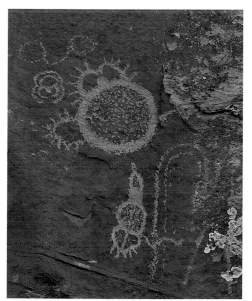 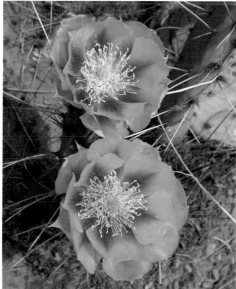

*We'll never know what the petroglyph artists had in mind when they incised images like these, but maybe they were inspired by the great nature around them, such as these cactus in bloom.*

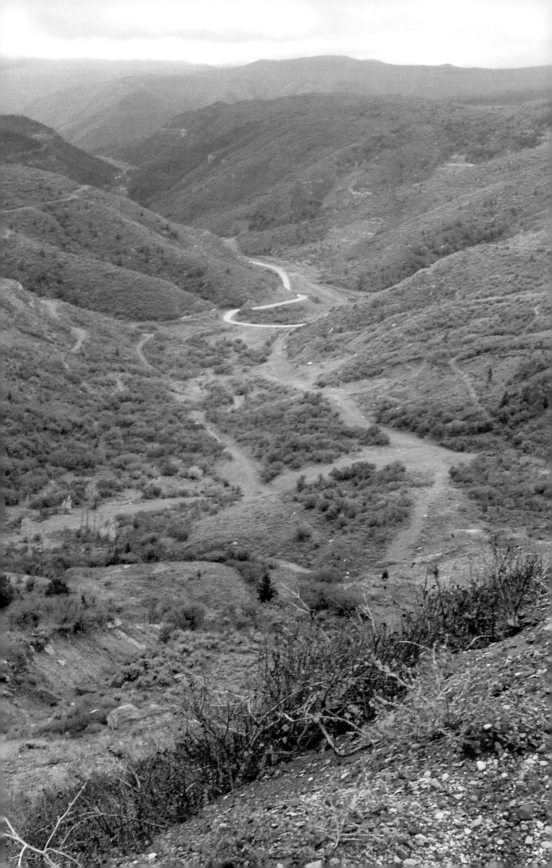

# DOUGLAS PASS FOSSIL SITE

## 13

**Directions:** Douglas Pass is about half-way between Rangely and Loma on CO 139. At the apex of the pass follow the gravel road which passes uphill to the left of the highway department depot. Stay on the main road. In about 5 miles you will come to a gate for the FAA station. Do NOT enter this property, it is a posted federal restricted area. Park well down from the gate, and walk uphill perpendicular to the road. You will encounter shallow pits in the fossil beds. Be sure to keep well away from the FAA area lest you end up taking a shortcut to Guantanamo Bay.

**Contact Info:**
there is no contact info for this site as it is not improved or maintained

**Fee:** no fee

**Hours:** year-round daylight hours

**Best time to visit:** summer is the ticket here as the elevation allows you respite from the heat below

**Camping/Lodging:** basic camping on BLM lands nearby; nearest lodging is in Fruita

**Access:** moderate both in driving and hiking; the altitude can have an effect on you here—pay attention to it; don't attempt this site in bad weather

**Jon's Rating:** ★★★☆☆ (paleontology)

**Jon's Notes:**
As mountain trails go Douglas Pass—at a bit over 8,000 feet—is not much to brag about, but that's good news for you because during most of the summer the area is snow-free. Yet don't be fooled, at times it can still get mighty cold up there, even in the middle of July. As you drive up the dirt road from the pavement of CO 139 you'll notice the peaks surrounding you are not the typical hard rock granites of the Rocky Mountains but are actually soft layered shales of the Green River Formation. These sediments accumulated in giant freshwater lakes during the Eocene Epoch, some 55 million (plus or minus a few hundred thousand) years ago. This region was more tropical back then, a story told by the fossils found here, including fronds of palm trees, zillions of insects and fish.

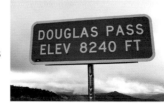

*LEFT: If nothing else, Douglas Pass is a scenic drive on the way to Dinosaur National Monument.*

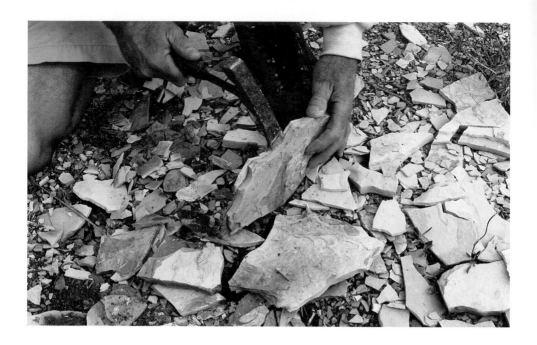

*ABOVE: The fossils here are trapped in fine layers of shale. It's all about splitting apart the rock to reveal the fossils within*

*RIGHT: Some of the fossils at Douglas Pass are exquisite.*

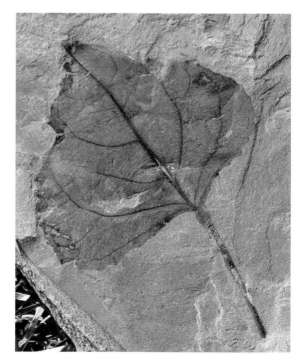

## INVERTEBRATES RULE!

It's a sad fact that there's not many places where a fossil enthusiast like you can look for—that is, dig for—fossils on public land. The highly political "Fossil Wars" of the 20th century have spilled over into the 21st and you need to know that you are not allowed to collect fossils of vertebrates (animals with backbones) from public land without a permit. And unless you are affiliated with a museum or educational institution, said permit will not be forthcoming. However, the BLM publishes a little brochure on the rules it has adopted lately called "Fossils on America's Public Lands" and in it you'll find that collecting reasonable amounts of fossil invertebrates and plants for personal use is allowed on BLM land. The good news is 99% of the fossils at Douglas Pass fall into these categories. Just keep in mind that "personal use" does not allow for selling them.

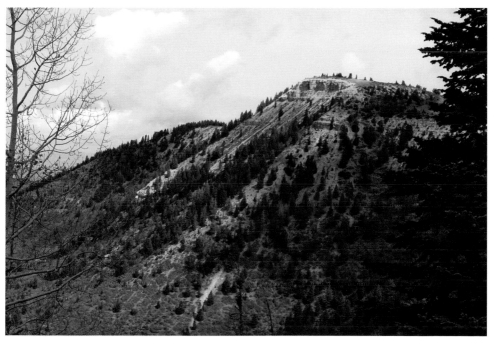

*The ancient shale splits along sedimentary bedding planes, revealing traces of life from 55 million years ago.*

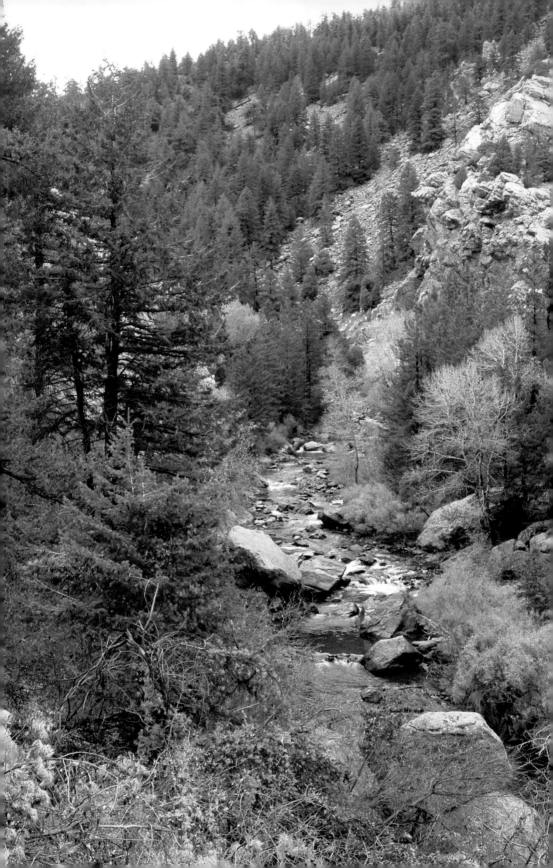

# ELDORADO CANYON STATE PARK

## 14

**Directions:** From Boulder follow CO 93 south about 5 miles to the turnoff for Eldorado Springs. The Visitor Center is about a mile up into the canyon but the most scenic aspect is before you get there.

**Contact Info:**
Eldorado Canyon State Park
303-494-3943
http://parks.state.co.us/Parks/eldoradocanyon

**Fee:** vehicle entrance fee

**Hours:** daylight hours

**Best time to visit:** mid-summer is great, but it's also got the masses, with hordes of climbers filling the parking areas before dawn; if you have a choice, go for mid-week in the fall; the turning leaves make for good photo ops and it's way less crowded

**Camping/Lodging:** improved camping nearby and lodging in Boulder

**Access:** easy–moderate–extreme; the drive is easy; the hiking is usually moderate but can be from easy–difficult; the rock climbing is superb—it's some of the best rock in the country; climbing routes at "Eldo" can get downright extreme with multiple pitches up to 5.13

**Jon's Rating:** ★★★☆☆ (geology)

**Jon's Notes:**
It comes as no surprise that the area around Boulder is loaded with picturesque scenery, being as it is situated at the base of the Front Range. Still, it astounds me the amazing beauty of some of the places which one can drive right up into. Along with its pristine cascading waterfalls and miles of excellent hiking trails, Eldorado Canyon is well-known as a rock climber's paradise. The variety of routes and hardened quartzite of its walls attract climbers from the world over to test their mettle in the vertical arena. You can travel through the central canyon just below the famous walls and watch the climbers do their thing while cooling your toes in the crystalline mountain stream. Just don't park along the roadside here, lest your car body ends up with an unwanted adjustment!

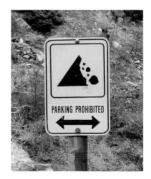

*LEFT: A quiet, picture-perfect mountain setting just minutes from Boulder.*

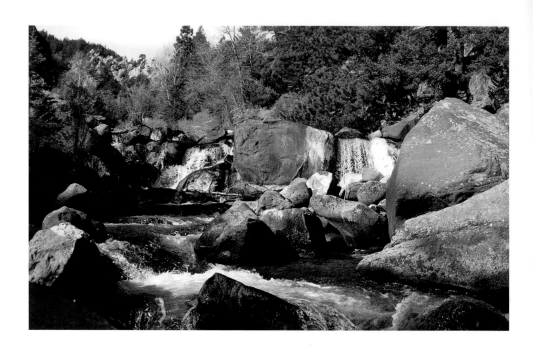

*A river runs through it. In this case it's clear, cold and soothing after a long hot summer day of climbing.*

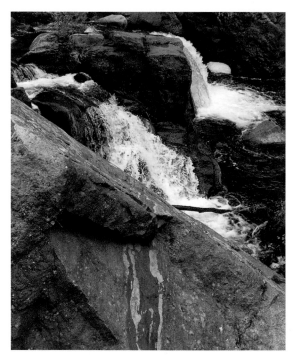

## THE RICHES OF ELDORADO

The promise of wealth and opportunity beckons from this legendary canyon. But it's not of the monetary kind. Rather, it's of the vertical sort. Eldorado is rich with climbing opportunity. The rock is hard, clean, quartzite and there's an unlimited variety of routes. When hiking along the trails below the cliffs, you are likely to see rock climbers dancing along the near-vertical walls above, having the time of their lives.

"That's crazy," you might say, depending on whether you're a climber or not. But stop and watch awhile. Examine the precision with which they climb. You'll see it's not the haphazard, reckless, dare-devil sport you might imagine. Climbers go in teams—usually two at a time—so as to belay (protect) one another as they climb. Although a bit extreme, this sport holds challenge and reward unlike any other.

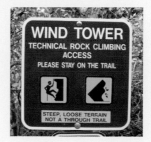

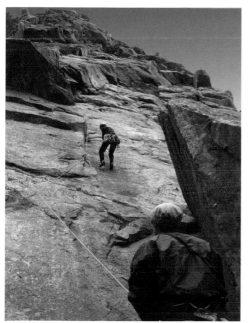

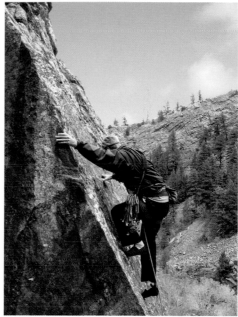

*Rock climbing on Wind Tower. It's safer than it looks if you know what you're doing.*

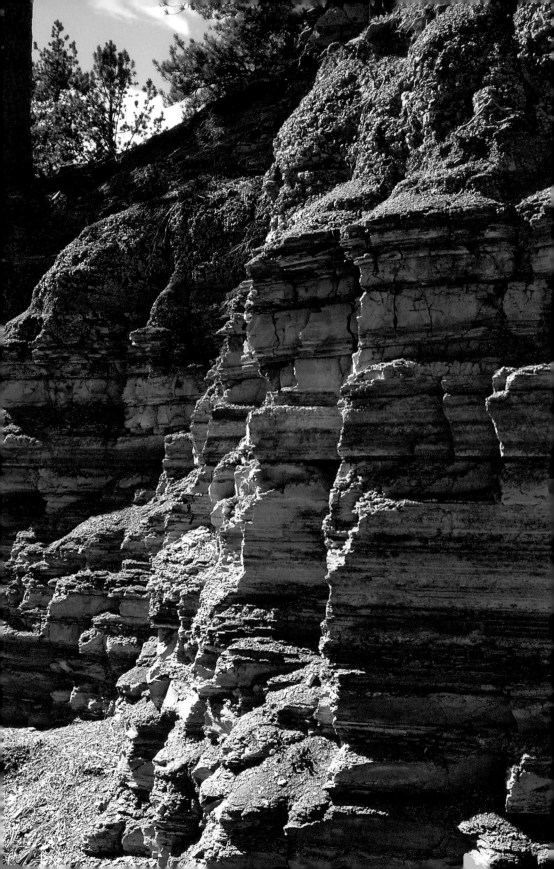

# FLORISSANT FOSSIL BEDS NATIONAL MONUMENT

## 15

**Directions:** The monument is just south of the little town of Florissant which is about 15 miles west of Divide on US 24. The private digging quarry is along the same road before you reach the monument.

**Contact Info:**
Florissant Fossil Beds National Monument
719-748-3253
www.nps.gov/flfo

**Fee:** fee area

**Hours:** the park is open year-round; visitor center hours are seasonal

**Best time to visit:** early summer through fall

**Camping/Lodging:** camping and lodging in Florissant

**Access:** easy; the big sequoia stumps are next to the visitor center

**Jon's Rating:** ★★★★☆ (paleontology)

**Jon's Notes:**
Once upon a time 35 million years ago, a series of volcanic eruptions spewed out a lot of ugly debris that clogged the local stream valley and consequently produced a lake. The nasty volcanoes kept at it by belching smoke and ash, asphyxiating and burying animals and plants of all sorts for uncountable centuries. Today the valley is filled in with these ancient sediments but its secret past has been revealed. The extra-fine layers produce extra-fine fossils including delicate butterflies with wing patterns and sequoia stumps the size of delivery trucks.

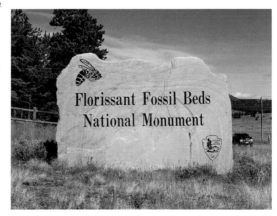

*LEFT: The fine "paper shales" of Florissant have preserved some of the finest fossils anywhere..*

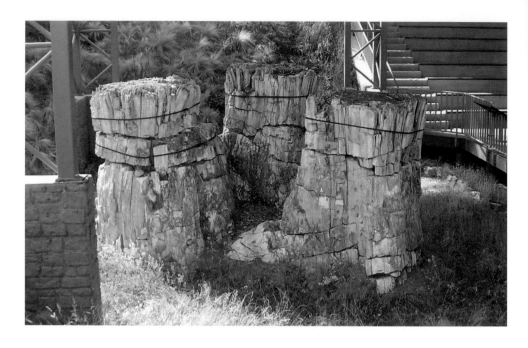

*This unsung gem of the National Park Service has been around awhile but sadly doesn't get enough attention from the government to install a proper museum or visitor center. Still, the giant fossilized sequoia stumps alone are worth the trek. Besides, it's only a short gallop from the wild west of Cripple Creek.*

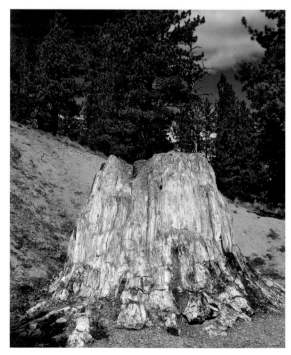

## DIG IT—BUT NOT HERE

Just because the Florissant Valley is public land over-flowing with incredible fossils does not mean you can dig holes willy-nilly wherever you please. The fact is you are not allowed to dig or collect fossils on Monument grounds. Period. Don't even think of it. Happily, however, you may dig your butt off just north of the monument at the Florissant Fossil Quarry (florissantfossils@earthlink.net). For a small fee you are outfitted with tools of the trade and are virtually guaranteed of finding fossils. The last time we visited, a "junior paleontologist" named Emily found a very rare and fantastic butterfly wing (see photo below).

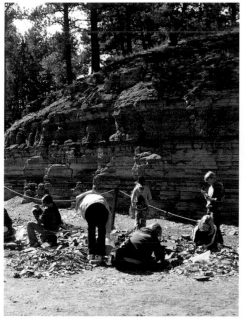 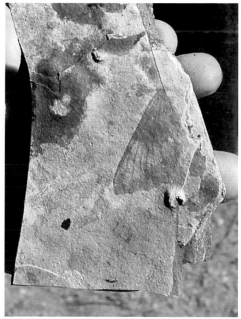

*It's pure luck—sometimes you find nothing but fossil leaf fragments all day long and then—BINGO!—you split open a rock and find a fossilized butterfly.*

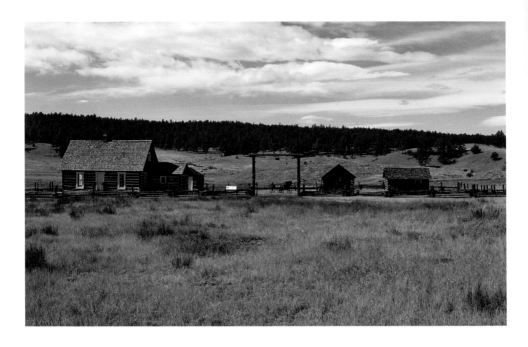

*It looks peaceful enough, that's why early pioneers settled here in the mid-1800s. Little did they know there was quite a Rock-and-Roll party here 35 million years ago!*

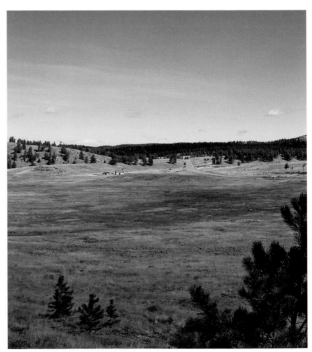

## PAPER SHALES

Fossils occur in all sorts of sediments from the sandy gravel of rivers to the fine muck of a northland bog. All things considered, as a general rule, the finer the sediment grains, the better may be preserved the details of a critter being buried. Florissant is renowned for its superb, very detailed fossils. The architects of it all were the volcanoes, which continually puffed out clouds of super-fine ash, entombing the plants and animals in delicate layers known as "paper shales." Some of the lamina are so fine they are no thicker than a sheet of paper.

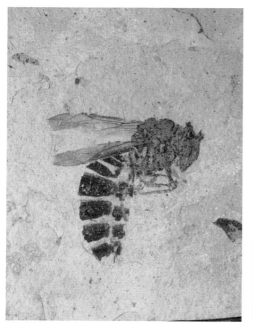 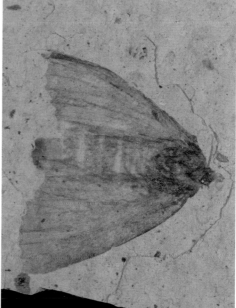

*The most fragile elements of life from 34 million years ago are preserved in these unique paper shales.*

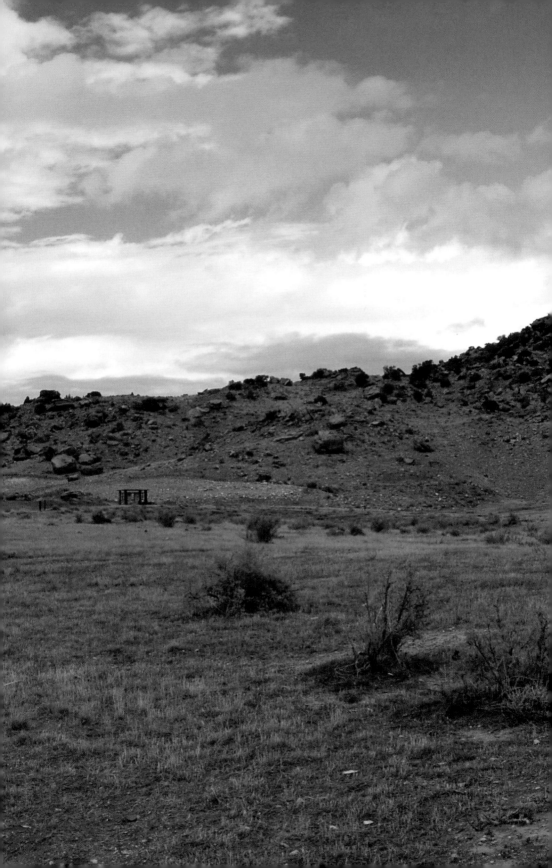

# FRUITA PALEO AREA

## 16

**Directions:** From Fruita take CO 340 south about 1 mile to west on Kings View (follow the signs for Horse Thief Canyon ). Pavement ends in 3/5 miles. The Fruita Paleo area is another 1½ miles further on the left.

**Contact Info:**
BLM Colorado
970-244-3000
www.dinosaurdiamond.org
www.co.blm.gov/mcnca
www.dinosaurjourney.org

**Fee:** no fee

**Hours:** year-round daylight hours

**Best time to visit:** anytime it's not raining or snowing

**Camping/Lodging:** improved camping and lodging in Fruita and Grand Junction

**Access:**
moderate; the parking area itself is a challenge to negotiate!

**Jon's Rating:** ★★★★★ (paleontology)

**Jon's Notes:**
The Fruita Paleo Area is a bold attempt to involve students, tourists, and everyday townsfolk in the science that brings long-dead things back to life. There's a hiking trail that flows through the pastel-colored sediments and signage along the way describing the ancient environments that each layer represents. Graphics do most of the work of recreating the scene and all you have to do is walk along and deal with the heat.

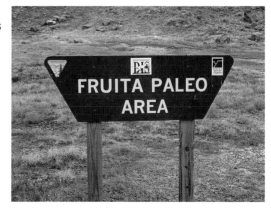

*LEFT: It looks like just a bunch of rocks, and it is, but . . .*

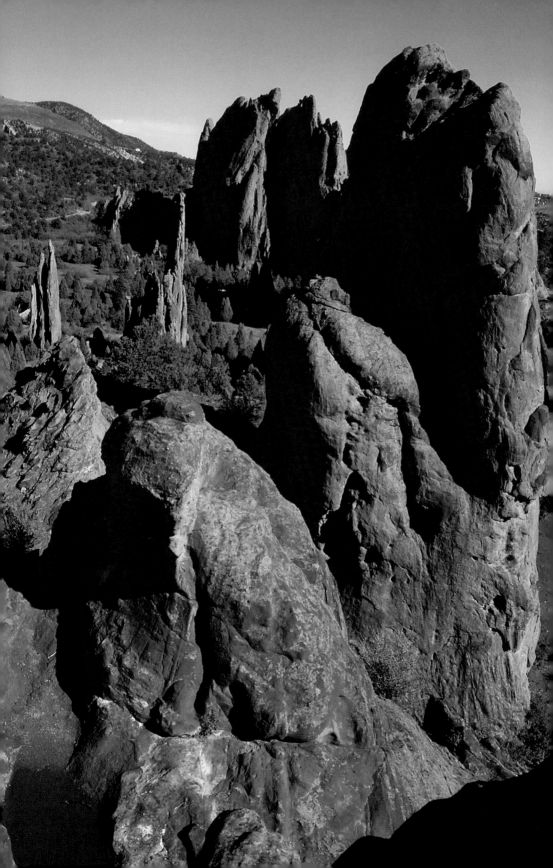

# GARDEN OF THE GODS

## 17

**Directions:** This park is in Colorado Springs. From I-25 follow Garden of the Gods Parkway west about 2 1/2 miles. Turn south (left) on 30th St. The visitor center is about 2 miles.

**Contact Info:**
Garden of the Gods
719-634-6666
www.gardenofgods.com

**Fee:** no fee

**Hours:** park: summer 5am–11pm, winter 5am–9pm; visitor center hours vary seasonally

**Best time to visit:** anytime you want to relax and get away from the grind is a good time to visit Garden of the Gods; this place is magical even in the rain

**Camping/Lodging:** improved camping and lodging in Colorado Springs

**Access:** easy to moderate; if you want extreme, get a rock climbing permit at the visitor center

**Jon's Rating:** ★★★★☆ (geology)

**Jon's Notes:**
Colorado Springs is growing so fast the highway department can't keep up with the traffic, a fact you'll no doubt enjoy if you find yourself stuck in a bumper-to-bumper crawl along I-25. But there is a remedy for those rush hour blues and Garden of the Gods is it. You can't help but feel calmed when you walk among the giant Mesozoic "hog-backs," as these tall, red slabs of conglomerate are called. The pathways weave in-and-out of impressive walls of up-turned strata while balanced rocks and erosional spires greet you in between. It's been a Native American spiritual place for ages and you too can find religion, practice transcendental meditation, sit in zazen, or just plain mellow out.

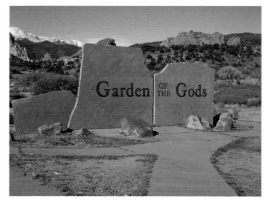

*LEFT: The Gods have a garden and you're invited into it.*

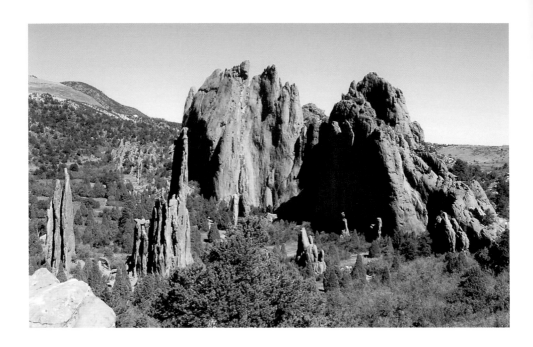

Don't ask me why,
but the giant slabs of
sandstone tilted up
on end here are
called "hog-backs."
It's one of those
geologic terms invent-
ed to confuse folks.
Oh, go ahead, look it
up in the glossary.

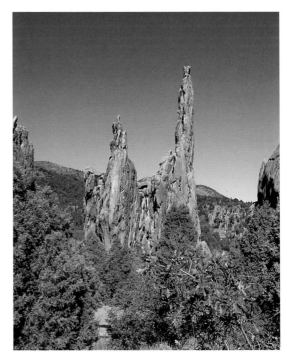

## PLAYING GOD IN THE GARDEN

The geology of Garden of the Gods is so impressive it looks out of place among the crowded flatlands of housing subdivisions and shopping complexes surrounding it. While mapping the geology here in the early 1980s, my friend George and I were constantly stopped by tourists in the park who wondered if the huge formations were really natural or had they "been made-up by some Hollywood movie director?" That, of course, was an invitation to elaborate on the pitfalls of shoddy workmanship and inferior materials used in various monuments back in the day, all-the-while feeding into the person's impression that these were, in fact, very large props. After sufficient discourse we'd reveal the truth and they'd leave—either more confused or more impressed, but hopefully a little better educated in geology. They certainly didn't seek our counsel any more after that.

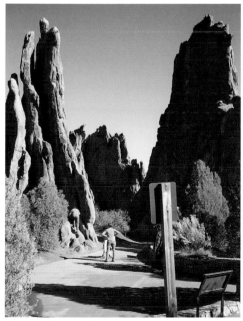

*Almost every view is a photo op.*

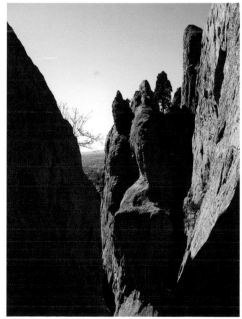

*View along some of the famous "hog-backs."*

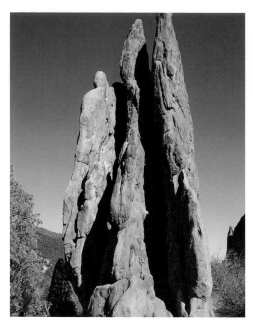

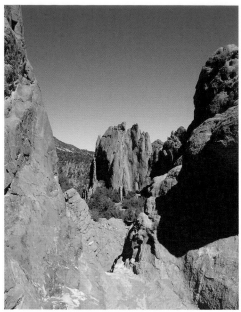

As you might imagine, this is a climber's dreamland. Climbers here are afforded special status, being allowed access to many areas where the public cannot go. Routes with varying degrees of difficulty are found among the crags and spires.

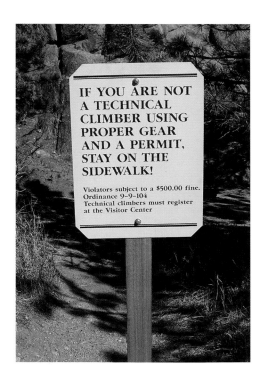

IF YOU ARE NOT A TECHNICAL CLIMBER USING PROPER GEAR AND A PERMIT, STAY ON THE SIDEWALK!

Violators subject to a $500.00 fine.
Ordinance 9-9-104
Technical climbers must register at the Visitor Center

## BOTTOMS-UP!

It may be obvious to some of you more astute geology buffs, but the rocks here are not easily explained. For convenience we'll skip the easy part when the original sandstone sediments formed in roughly horizontal layers many millions of years ago (like about 300 million, but who's counting? . . . ) Let's jump ahead a few hundred million years to the Cenozoic during the mountain-building episodes which formed the Rockies. Amid all the hubub of high pressure and tremendous forces, the original sandstone beds were twisted, bent and otherwise shown very little respect for their position. Ultimately they were up-ended, resulting in slabs that are not just vertical, they're over-turned—which means the upper part is actually the bottom. Selective weathering did the rest.

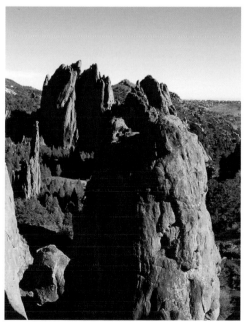
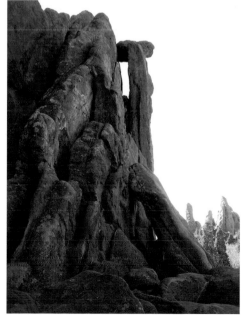

*Things get a bit mixed up here geologically speaking—if you want to find the top of the sandstone beds, look at the bottom.*

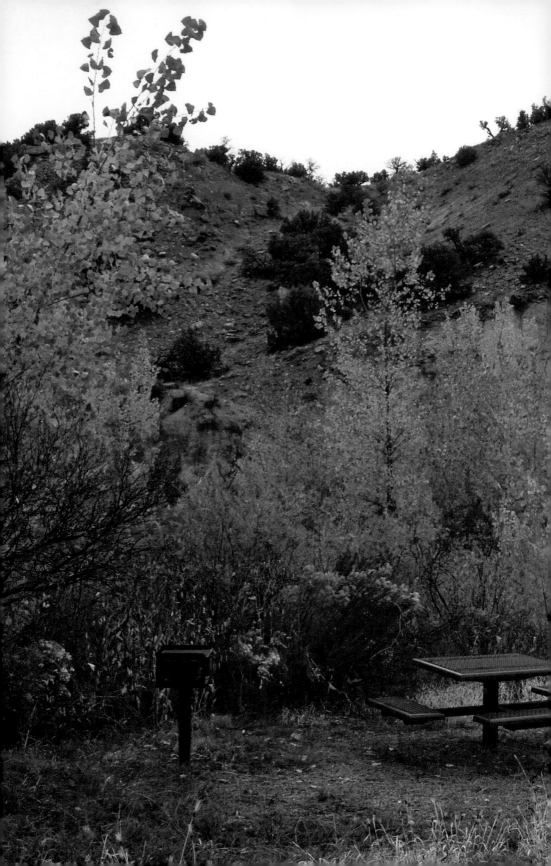

**Directions:** It's not the easiest trying to find Red Canyon Rd. but that's what you want to be on north of Cañon City. Once you find it, Garden Park is about 4⁴/₅ miles north of town. There's a picnic area, pit toilet and signs.

**Contact Info:**
Dinosaur Depot
800-987-6379
www.dinosaurdepot.com

**Fee:** no fee

**Hours:** year-round daylight hours

**Best time to visit:** fall is the most enjoyable with the colorful foliage adding to the otherwise static displays

**Camping/Lodging:** camping and lodging in Cañon City

**Access:** easy paved trail

**Jon's Rating:** ★★★★★ (paleontology)

**Jon's Notes:**
When you visit Garden Park there's probably not gonna be a lot to see in the way of dinosaurs but this area has produced some of the finest specimens of the science. In the 1870s amateur paleontologists from Cañon City discovered giant fossil bones along Fourmile Creek, touching off a "dinosaur rush" to the region similar to that of the popular gold rushes, albeit on a much smaller scale. Periodically, bones are still found in the area. You can learn more about it and see some of the incredible finds at the Dinosaur Depot in town.

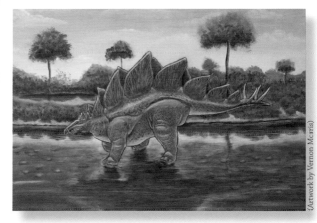

(Artwork by Vernon Morris)

*LEFT: They were once here, but now they're gone (again). Too bad because now this place is not much more than a nice place to stroll along the creek.*

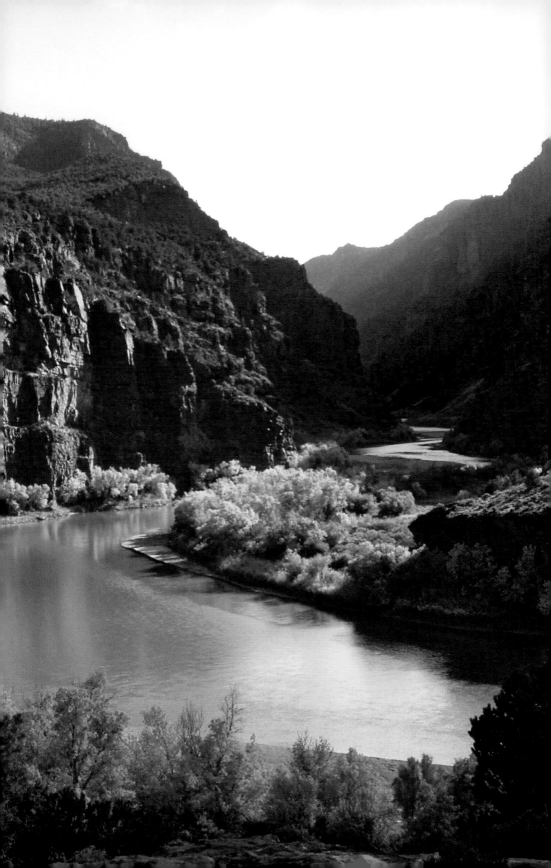

# GATES OF LODORE

**Directions:** The "Gates" are just inside the northern section of Dinosaur National Monument. From Maybell, travel northwest on CO 318 approximately 40 miles. Turn left on county 10 and then right on county 34. Follow the signs and you'll be in the park at the end of the road in about 10 miles. The Gates of Lodore await you there.

**Contact Info:**
Dinosaur National Monument
970-374-3000
www.nps.gov/dino

**Fee:** entrance fee

**Hours:** year-round

**Best time to visit:** fall is the most beautiful and also the least crowded of the nice weather months

**Camping/Lodging:** improved camping at the park; nearest lodging is in Craig

**Access:** easy–moderate; or, for a real adventure, go rafting!

**Jon's Rating:** ★★★✦☆ (geology)

**Jon's Notes:**
Aptly named, the Gates of Lodore are imposing rock buttresses which flank the entrance to Lodore Canyon and the great canyons of the Green River as it courses through Dinosaur National Monument. At some points the canyons are over 3000' deep. The "Gates" themselves loom large and imposing, giving you a sense of foreboding as you enter the canyons, especially if you're on a raft. But, hey, you don't have to worry about it if you view the Gates from the trail at the campground near them. You'll be safely ¼ mile away, out of reach of the giant Cyclops and other monsters which may dwell within.

*LEFT: It sounds foreboding—The Gates of Lodore—but it's not too bad once you slay the dragon around the corner . . .*

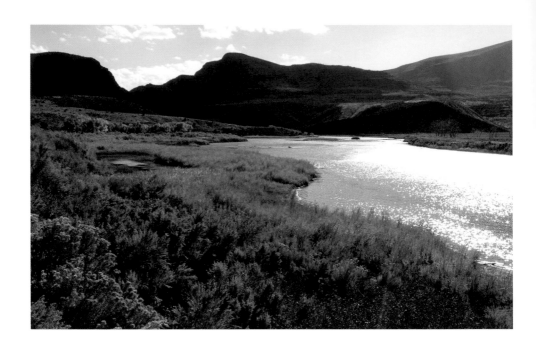

The Green River in fall spectacle, just before the Gates.

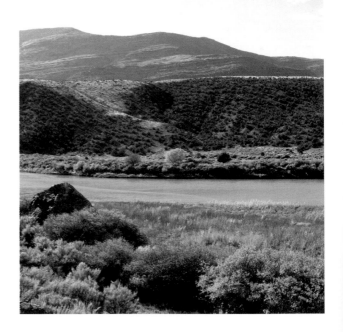

## FALL IN

Fall 'tis the season to be jolly here as the multiple hues of autumn give an artistic touch to the landscape with a rich pallet of colors. September and October are the best times with very few people, cool weather and beautiful scenery. For an especially wonderful adventure, sign up for a rafting trip down the Green River. It's not wild like the Grand Canyon, but it's just as thrilling. Contact outfitters in Vernal.

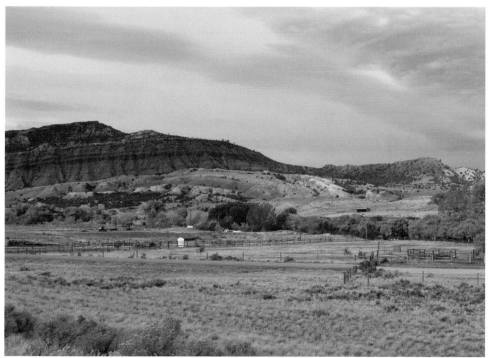

*Even outside the Gates it's a kaleidoscope of color.*

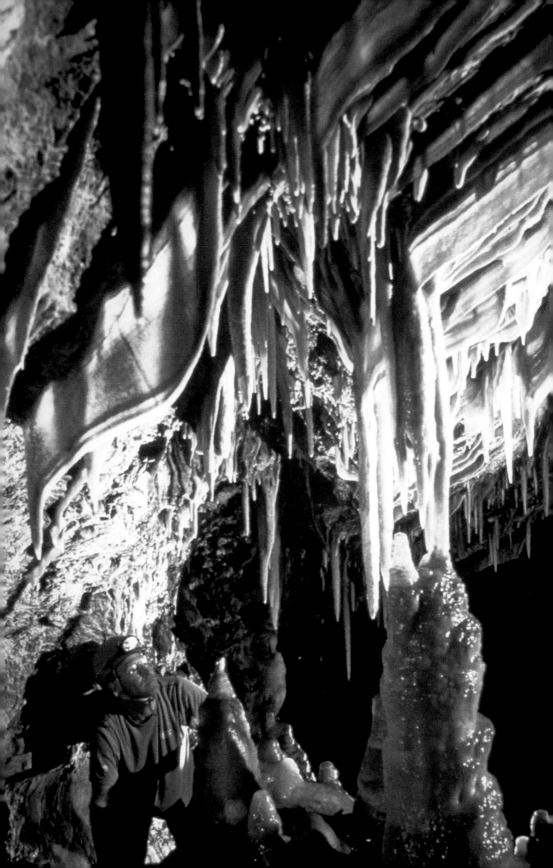

# GLENWOOD CAVERNS AND GLENWOOD HOT SPRINGS

**Directions:** Both of these places are in Glenwood north of I-70. The Caverns are slightly northwest of town at 5100 Two Rivers Plaza Rd. The Pool is right in town at 401 N. River St. Signs direct you to both once you're off the interstate.

**Contact Info:**
Glenwood Caverns Adventure Park
800-530-1635
www.glenwoodcaverns.com

Hot Springs Pool
800-537-7946
www.hotspringspool.com

**Fee:** entrance and user fee for both

**Hours:** cavern 9:30am–8pm daily; pool 7:30am–10pm daily

**Best time to visit:** a visit to the hot springs on a snowy day is way cool—I mean warm—but you can enjoy it just as well anytime you get there; the caverns are pretty much the same every day

**Camping/Lodging:** improved camping and lodging in town

**Access:** super easy access for the pool; there's 127 steps going down into the cave, but once you navigate that it's a fairly easy tour on maintained paths

**Jon's Rating:** ★★★★☆ (geology)

**Jon's Notes:**
It's almost too much to ask for—the biggest and best hot springs of Colorado AND the biggest and best caverns of Colorado, both in the same place. Geologically it's mere coincidence that these two "best-of" sites are here in the same town but you're the better for it, especially if you can hang around town for awhile. The caverns will impress you underground, while the hot spring pools will impress and relax you above. The atmosphere is Colorado grandeur both above and below and there's plenty of room, especially in the HUGE spring pool, to spread out and keep to yourself.

*LEFT: There's a reason this is Colorado's premier underground experience. Actually, there are several reasons . . .*

## GET DOWN UNDERGROUND

If you take the almost-a-mile-long Iron Mountain Tramway to reach the cave entrance, you can't help but think that a gondola ride through the stratosphere is a most unique, if ironic, way to begin a cavern tour. Once you get to the entrance you've got to trudge down over 120 steps before you even really begin your underground adventure, so be ready to get-down underground. Once inside you'll see why this place attracts visitors from around the world on a regular basis and is also the defacto base of operations for the Colorado Grotto of the NSS (National Speleological Society).

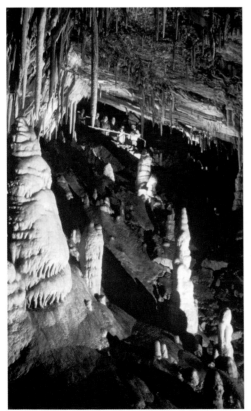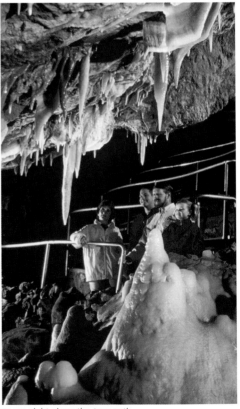

*Some of the best speleothems (cave formations) in the state are right along the tour path.*

## THE COLORADO WARM-UP

When we said in the description this was the biggest hot springs in Colorado what we actually meant is it's the largest hot springs facility in the entire U.S. It's stature as such is attributable not only by virtue of it's humongous pool (larger than a football field holding over 1 million gallons!), but also its outflow—a whopping 3.5 million gallons a day. There are two pools—the big one is kept at about 90 degrees, the small one at about 104.

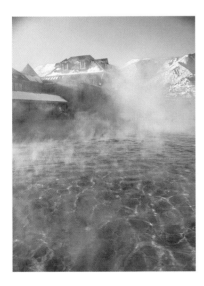

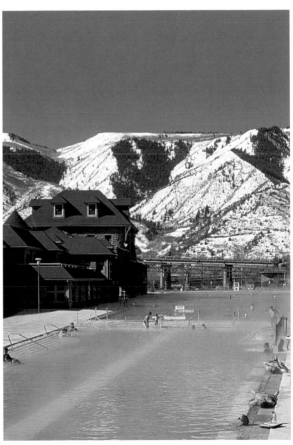

*After your cool-down underground, how about a warm-up in the hot springs? One of America's greatest hot springs is right in town. There's plenty of room for everyone in the million-gallon pool and you can't beat the view!*

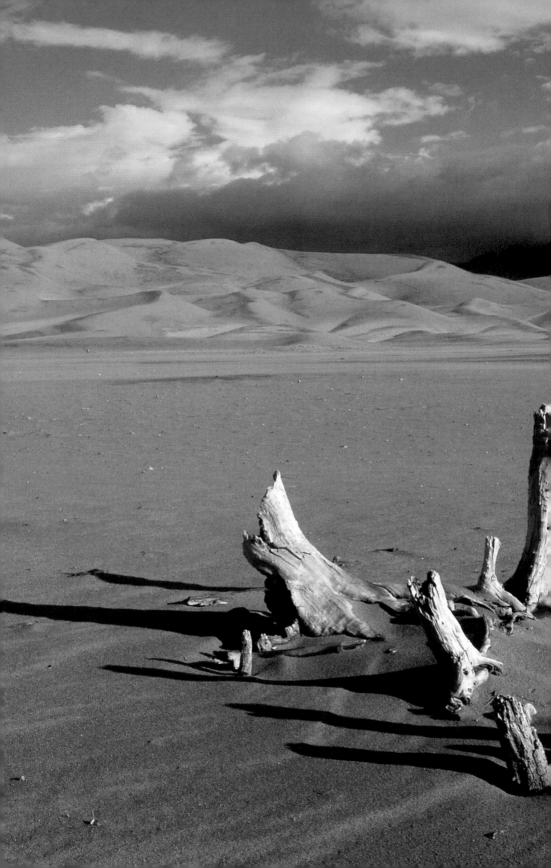

# GREAT SAND DUNES NATIONAL PARK

## 21

**Directions:** From Alamosa head east on US 160. In 14 miles turn north on CO 150. The Visitor Center is about 16 miles. Look for the giant pile of sand.

**Contact Info:**
Great Sand Dunes National Park
719-378-6300
www.nps.gov/grsa

**Fee:** vehicle entrance fee

**Hours:** park open year-round; visitor center hours are seasonal

**Best time to visit:** avoid the really hot days of mid-summer, unless, of course, you want a true taste of that roasting-your-sorry-butt-in-the-desert experience

**Camping/Lodging:** improved camping in park; nearest lodging in Alamosa

**Access:** easy–difficult; if the wind is blowing stronger than 20 mph then do yourself a favor and stay inside at the visitor center

**Jon's Rating:** ★★★★☆ (geology)

**Jon's Notes:**
There's more than a few folks who buy the Guinness Book of World Records, searching the voluminous pages of minutiae for the biggest ball of twine, the tallest stack of oil cans, or the greatest collection of Cabbage Patch dolls. If you're one of those type, and you've scoured the continent looking for the largest pile of sand, then you're in luck—this is it. More good news: they have a great visitor center and lots of interpretive trails so even if you are enslaved by trivia mania, you'll still enjoy this wonderland of sand which somehow brings out the kid in all of us. This place is especially dramatic at sunrise and sunset. If you camp here be sure to get one of the sites overlooking the dunes—it's indescribable.

*LEFT: One of the greatest active sand dune environments in North America.*

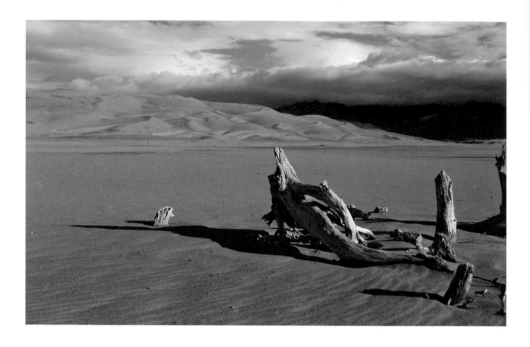

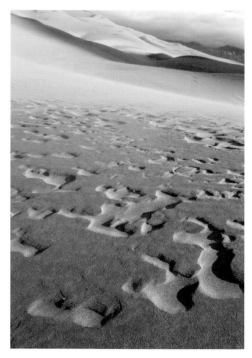

*Sand deserts are a dynamic environment, always changing, never the same from one minute to the next.*

*ABOVE: Skeleton of a lonesome tree trapped in the sand.*

*RIGHT: Mini dunes migrating over the surface of larger dunes. If you took a photo at this exact place 5 minutes later, you wouldn't recognize the spot.*

## ERGS?

What's the big deal about sand piles in the middle of Colorado? It's not like sand is rare or anything . . . Yet, when you get right down to the nitty gritty, such accumulations of sand—known as "ergs"—actually are uncommon. There's only a handful of such places in North America (Nevada, Arizona, Death Valley of California, as well as a few others) and most don't compare with this one. The dunes here reach an astonishing 700' in height above the valley and they are constantly shifting, a fact you'll take special notice of if you walk out here on a windy day. The area appears desolate but there's a surprisingly dynamic environment whose inhabitants and visitors live in harmony within the wilderness of grit.

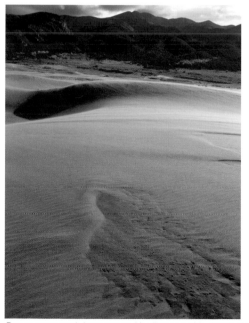 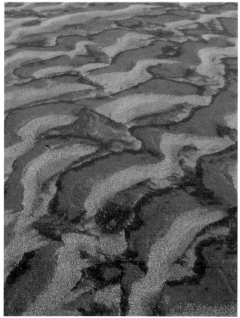

*Dunes come and dunes go and it all starts with simple ripples such as these (right).*

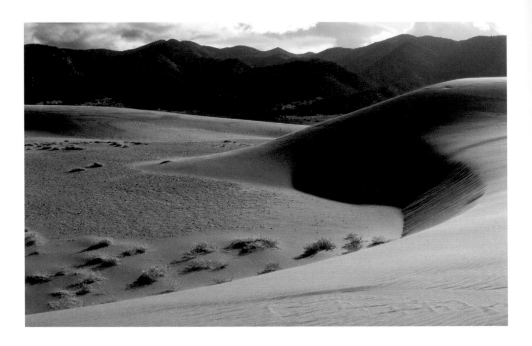

*This place somehow makes you just want to take off your shoes and run wild all day. Go ahead! Just don't forget to pick them up again later or they'll be quickly buried.*

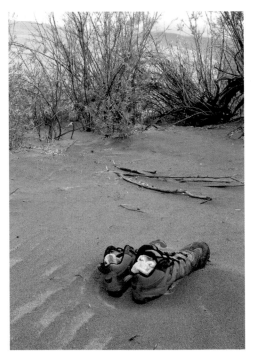

## TEXTURE AND SHADOW

The subtle shadows and textures found in dune environments are ever-changing and make for challenging study by artists and photographers alike. The nice thing about Great Sand Dunes is the color of the sands—various shades of brown and tan—simply because they are not white. This fact is appreciated among photographers because it minimizes the threat of overexposure which plagues areas with bleached-white sand. Here one is afforded interesting, workable, photogenic compositions throughout the day, even more so when there are a few clouds.

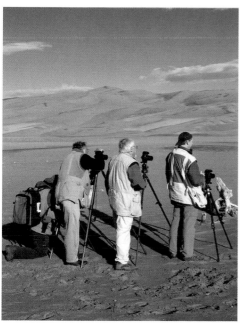
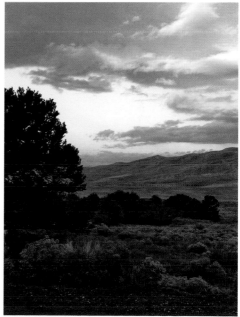

*The dramatic interplay of color, light and texture make this a photography classroom extraordinaire.*

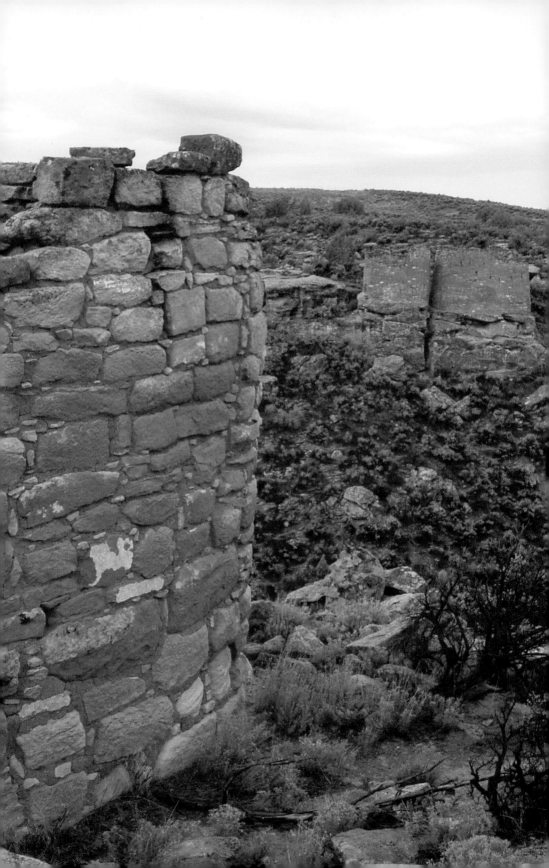

# HOVENWEEP NATIONAL MONUMENT

## 22

**Directions:** There are some sections of Hovenweep in Colorado but the best single part is just across the border in Utah at the visitor center. From Cortez head west on G Rd into Utah. About 3²/₅ miles after the state line turn north on Belitso Rd. (aka 401 Rd., aka Rt 2422) which bends to the west. In about 5 miles turn northeast on Reservation Rd (aka 413 Rd., aka Rt 2416). The visitor center is about 10 miles. You may also reach it from Painted Hands Pueblo in Canyons of the Ancients simply by following the paved road from there about 10 miles southwest.

**Contact Info:**
Hovenweep National Monument
970-562-4282
www.nps.gov/hove

**Fee:** per person entrance fee

**Hours:** park open year-round; visitor center hours are seasonal

**Best time to visit:** whenever the weather isn't sleeting or snowing; avoid the mid-summer heat waves

**Camping/Lodging:** improved camping at campground next to visitor center; closest lodging is in Cortez

**Access:** easy–moderate; the hike at the visitor center is fairly easy on maintained trails; exploring the outer areas are moderate–difficult

**Jon's Rating:** ★★★★★ (archaeology)

**Jon's Notes:**
A large part of this monument—including the visitor center—resides in Utah but it's literally right-next-door so if you're in the area you have to visit. Although it's not the law, if you pass this place up it will be a crime! The main complex of ruins abide along an incredible self-guided tour next to the visitor center called the Square Tower Ruins Trail. Although the canyon around which the trail winds is fairly small, it will defy your observation skills to try and pick out all the ruins— there's several dozen, many in superb condition.

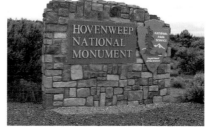

*LEFT: Rooms with a view . . .*

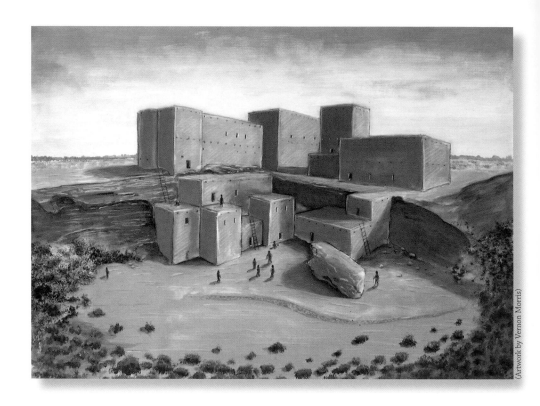

(Artwork by Vernon Morris)

Hovenweep has an extraordinary collection of fine buildings, some of which span several stories.

ABOVE: Artist reconstruction of Hovenweep Castle, back in the day. What a fine structure it was!

RIGHT: Hovenweep Castle as it is today.

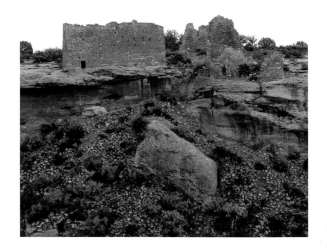

## MASONS IN THE LODGE

Despite all the hoopla, the Freemasons weren't the first architects of stonework in the Americas. The native Indians were. A trip around the ruins of Hovenweep will convince you these folks were not only accomplished builders, but true artisans. Hand-hewn rocks were fitted together in such precision that there was scarce need for mortar. As a result many of these structures are still somewhat standing, despite their centuries of exposure to weathering elements and looting by morons before the monument came along.

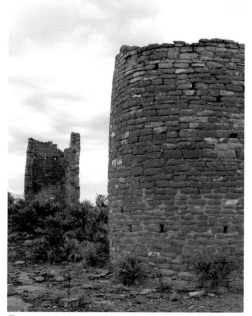
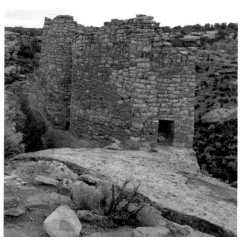

*They sure don't make things like they used to . . .*

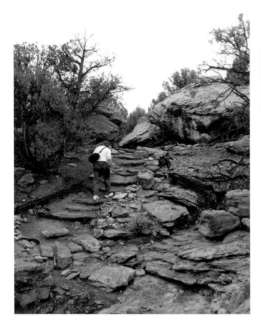

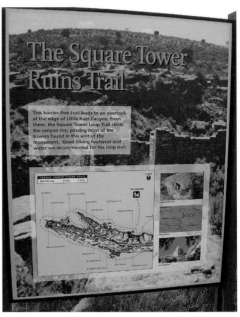

The trails are improved and you can complete the whole tour in less than 2 hours if you're pressed for time, which you shouldn't be if you visit this incredible canyon.

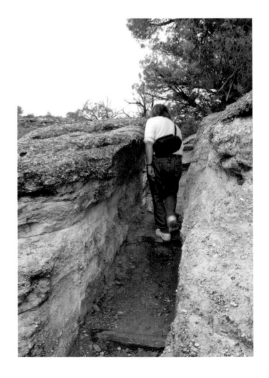

## DESERTED VALLEY

The term "Hovenweep" is a Ute word meaning "deserted valley." It was first applied by the pioneer photographer William Henry Jackson who visited the area in 1874. Ancestral Puebloan peoples first entered the area about A.D. 500 but took it easy for the first millennium. About A.D. 1150 eager developers cranked up the civic pride and began a building spree that carried on for a century. By the late 1200s, however, the rains had backed off and the region became more arid, prompting a move to greener pastures southwest.

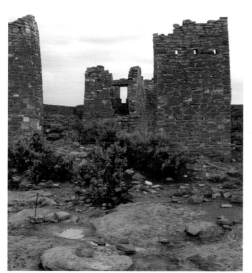
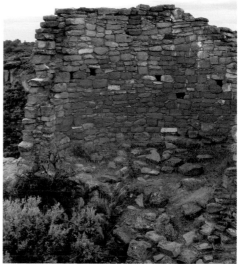

*It must have been hard for the ancients to decide they must leave this spectacular place.*

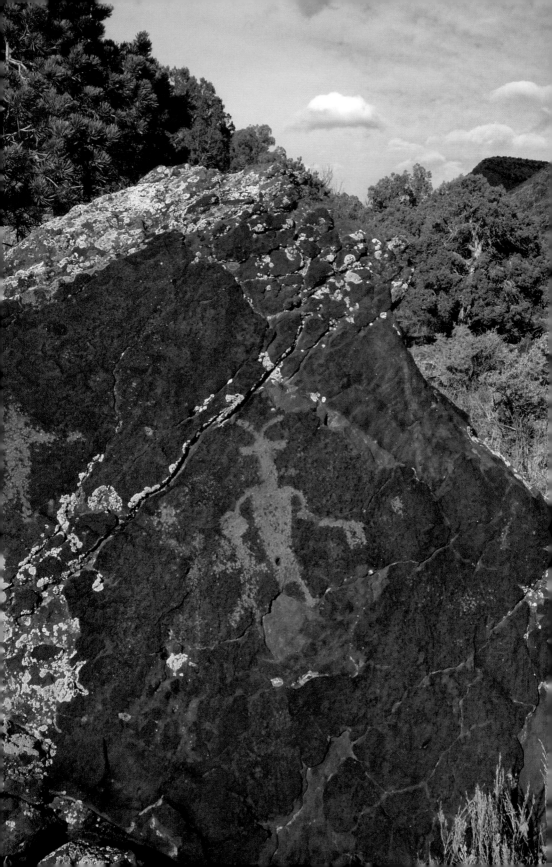

# IRISH CANYON

## 23

**Directions:** This canyon is located south of the Gates of Lodore, about 41 miles from Maybell. Whether traveling from the Gates of Lodore or Maybell, watch for mile marker 19 on CO 318. Turn north on county 10 and drive 4 miles to the interpretive station on your right. The petroglyphs occur on only 2 boulders—one on each side of the canyon entrance.

**Contact Info:**
Colorado BLM, Little Snake Field Office
970-826-5000
www.co.blm.gov/lsra/irishcanyon.htm

**Fee:** no fee

**Hours:** year-round daylight hours

**Best time to visit:** on your way to or from Gates of Lodore

**Camping/Lodging:** basic camping in the canyon; nearest lodging is in Craig

**Access:** easy—there's no way around it

**Jon's Rating:** ★★☆☆☆ (geology)
★☆☆☆☆ (archaeology)

**Jon's Notes:**
There's not a lot to it but if you're hankering for rock art, it's the only accessible spot in the immediate area. The most interesting thing about this site is the petroglyphs abide only on two rocks—one on

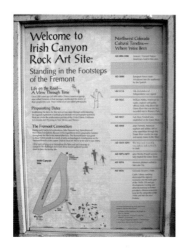

each side of the canyon entrance—a rare occurrence to say the least. Rock art often flanks the entrance to canyons, but when there's one, there's usually many more. Usually, but not here. After visiting the rock art site, take a drive into the canyon. It's pretty cool geologically speaking.

*LEFT: Usually there's more, but not here.*

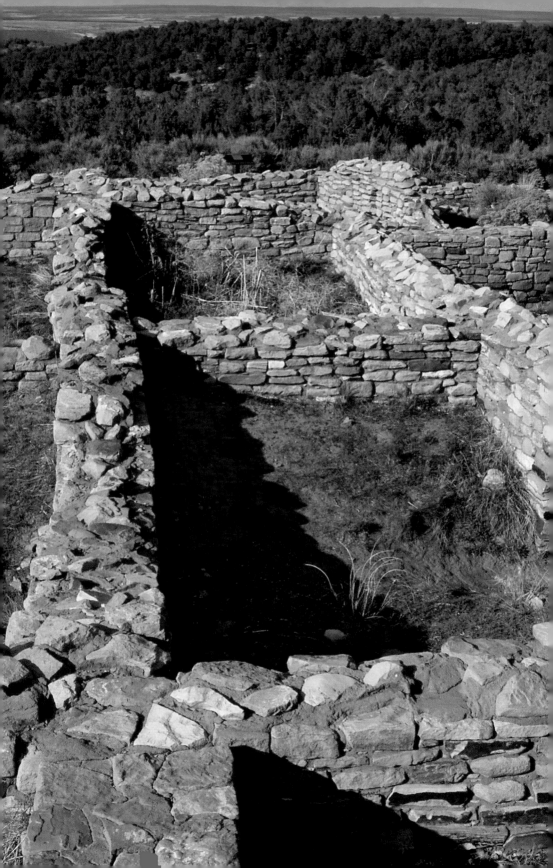

# LOWRY PUEBLO

## 24

**Directions:** This site is in the Canyons of the Ancients National Monument. From Anasazi Heritage Center head west on CO 184 to US 491. Drive north $9^2/5$ miles. At mile marker 46 turn west on Road CC. Follow for about $8^3/10$ miles and turn left onto—believe it or not—Rd 7.25. The ruins are about half a mile.

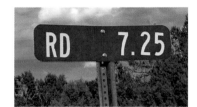

**Contact Info:**
Anasazi Heritage Center
970-882-4811
www.co.blm.gov/ahc/hmepge.htm

**Fee:** no fee to see the ruins; museum at heritage center has a modest entrance fee and it's worth it!

**Hours:** year-round daylight hours

**Best time to visit:** anytime; the road is good and the walk short

**Camping/Lodging:** basic camping on BLM land for free, but not in, or next to, any ruins; nearest lodging in Cortez

**Access:** easy and accessible

**Jon's Rating:** ★★★★☆ (archaeology)

**Jon's Notes:**
If you had any doubt about the quality of masonry construction in the 12th Century, Lowry Pueblo will help put your mind at ease. It is truly amazing how the locals got together, found all those rocks, and then stacked and cemented them so precisely. The walls are more square and vertical than most houses in my neighborhood today! Most of the pueblo has been stabilized in one fashion or another and you are permitted access to many of the rooms. A good time was had by all.

*LEFT: The pueblo with the most rooms in the immediate area.*

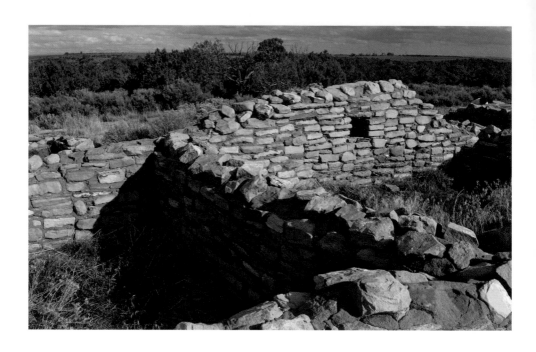

The walls of the pueblo have been stabilized and, as a result, you're allowed to access many of the dwellings.

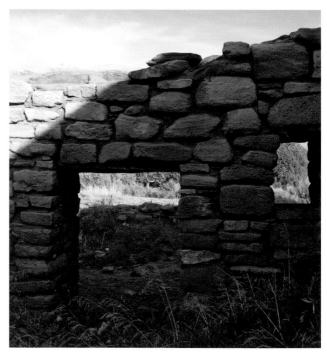

## THE BIG KAHUNA

The region surrounding Lowry Pueblo was littered with small communities when the Great House was in its heyday during the 12th Century. Archaeologists have discovered more than a hundred sites in the area, ranging from small pueblos to family units. Apparently, Lowry Pueblo was the Big Kahuna for the whole area which would account for not only its size and stature, but also its longevity. If you lived in the surrounding communities back then the chances are you would never have been invited into the Great House. But now you can laugh at history's foibles as you stride through the front door with impunity—if there is a front door.

(Artwork by Vernon Morris)

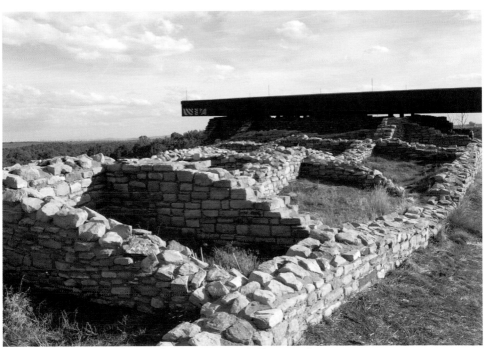

*Quality construction still holds even after the warranty period has expired.*

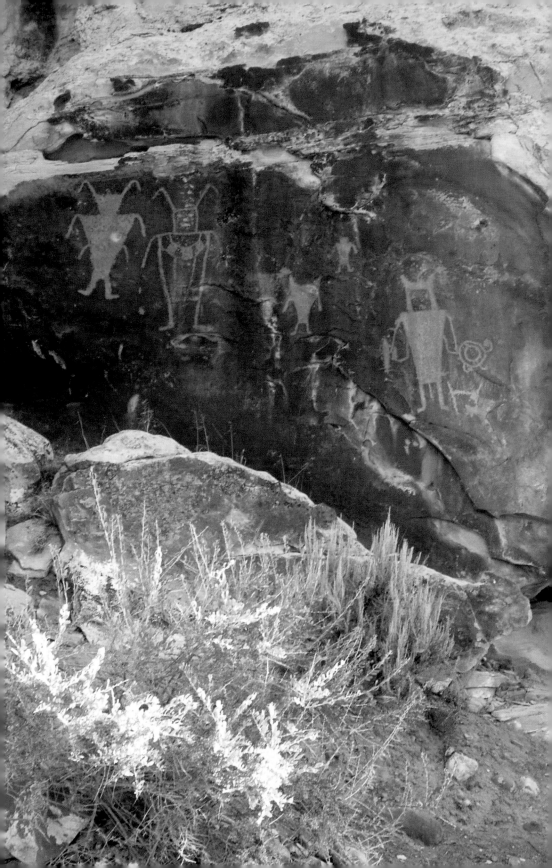

**Directions:** This site is part of Dinosaur National Monument and is actually in Utah. From Jensen, UT follow UT 149 north toward the monument visitor center. At about 2¹/₂ miles turn west onto Brush Creek Rd. In 4¹/₂ miles turn north on Island Park Rd. which eventually bends east. In approximately 15 miles you will enter Dinosaur National Monument. About ⁷/₁₀ miles after the border, look to the left up near the top of the mesa for the petroglyphs. If you get to the turnoff for Rainbow Park you've gone about a mile too far.

**Contact Info:**
Dinosaur National Monument
970-374-3000
www.nps.gov/dino

**Fee:** vehicle entrance fee to monument

**Hours:** year-round

**Best time to visit:** anytime you can get here, period

**Camping/Lodging:** campgrounds within the park; nearest lodging in Dinosaur

**Access:** easy–moderate; you can easily see the petroglyphs from the car with binoculars or you can hike up the slope to see them more closely; if you get up-close please do not touch the panels

**Jon's Rating:** ★★★★✦ (archaeology)

**Jon's Info:**
Some of the best petroglyphs in North America are also right next to the road. Such is the case here where the ultra-famous "anthropo-morph holding a sun" resides on the upper canyon wall along with a host of other very excellent and very precise images. Many of the images are clearly human-like and have been described as Shamans wearing elaborate necklaces and carrying sacred objects. Such definition is pure speculation, however, as we cannot travel back in time to ask the artists what they meant by it all. Unless, of course, you know someone at Area 51 that has a time machine. In case you didn't know it already, this is a "Littering Prohibited" monument—as evidenced by an overabundance of signs along the roadways.

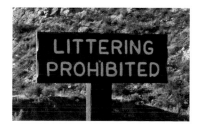

*LEFT: Some of the finest petroglyphs in North America are right here.*

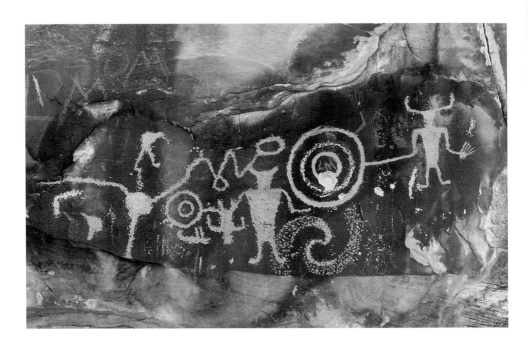

*Textbook examples of precision rock art right next to the road.*

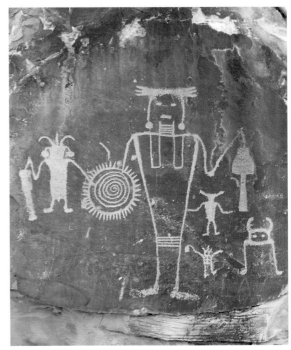

## PETROGLYPH 1-2-3

The petroglyph images are etched into sandstone which forms a protective cap rock above the softer sediments below it. The brown coating on the faces comes from iron oxides which have collected on the sandstone surface. Iron gets caught in solutions that percolate through the sandstone and once it reaches the surface, the iron precipitates and collects on the outside. After countless years, the outer edges become coated with a thick layer of rust-colored mineralization. When the artist pecks below the surface, the lighter contrasting color of the inner rock is revealed and—presto!—a petroglyph is born.

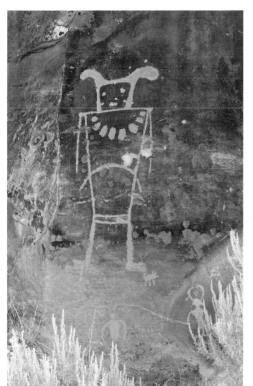

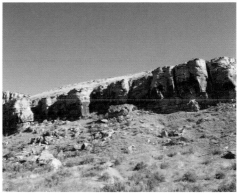

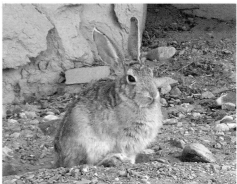

*It's a short hike up the hill to see the petroglyphs. Even Peter Rabbit was impressed!*

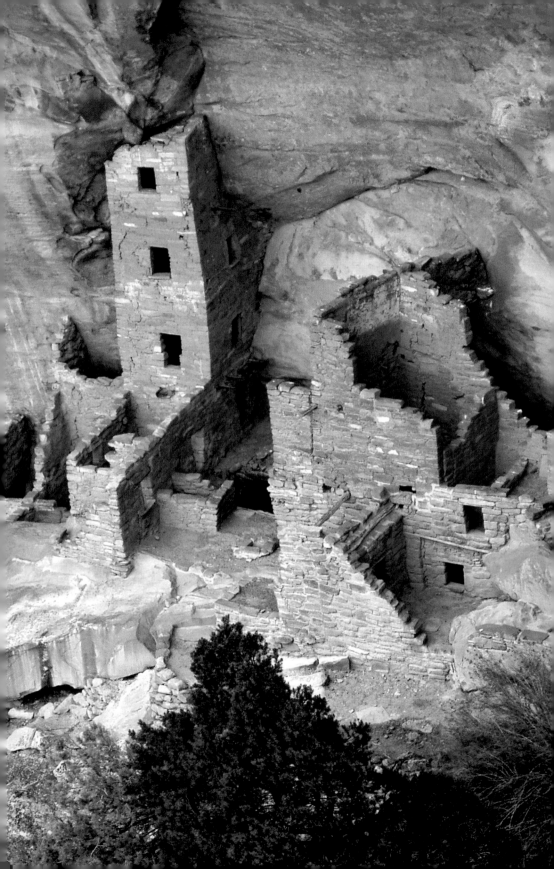

# MESA VERDE NATIONAL PARK

**Directions:** If you have a problem locating this famous site it's probably because you are in a foreign country and on another continent. Simply—Mesa Verde is about 9 miles east of Cortez and there's only one road in.

**Contact Info:**
Mesa Verde National Park
970-529-4465
www.nps.gov/meve

**Fee:** vehicle entrance fee

**Hours:** open year-round during daylight hours; roads around the mesa open at 7am; museum open 8am–5pm daily during summer season

**Best time to visit:** avoid the crowds by going in the off season and visiting the ruins early in the day; I like fall best.

**Camping/Lodging:** improved campgrounds and excellent lodging inside the park; these are closed in the winter

**Access:** easy–difficult; you can drive around and sample the overlooks or get adventurous by hiking routes such as the interesting Pictograph Trail

**Jon's Rating:** ★★★★★★ (archaeology)
★★★★★ (geology)

**Jon's Notes:**
About AD 600 some trendy suburbanites from the Four Corners region decided enough was enough. They canned their former free-wheeling nomadic lifestyle and took up a more sedentary life of farming and husbandry in the area around Chapin Mesa and Wetherill Mesa. These early settlers lived in simple pit houses scattered atop the mesas and in the valleys below. Over time, however, the town engineers developed more sophisticated structures built fully above ground. But then some know-it-all comes along—not content with living in a fancy pueblo—and starts building high-rises in the alcoves of the canyon walls. By 1200 the area's development boom was in full vigor. But you know how fickle the real estate biz can be! By 1300 all these structures were abandoned and the housing market collapsed.

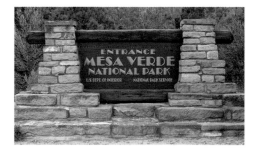

*LEFT: One of the most famous archaeological sites in the Southwest.*

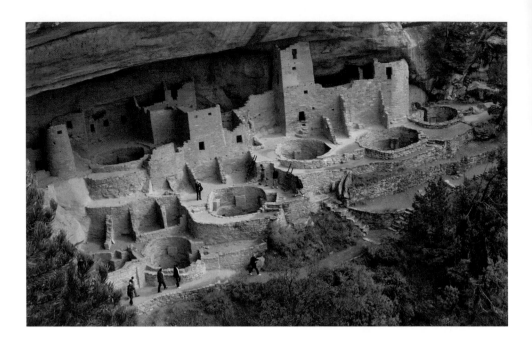

One of the most famous cliff dwellings in North America is aptly named Cliff Palace. The view from the overlook is stellar but it gets even better if you sign up for a guided tour.

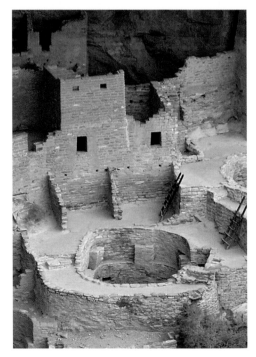

## CLIFF PALACE, ALL TO YOURSELF

If you're the type of person who appreciates spiritual places but only if it's quiet, then I assure you there are times when you'll go stark raving mad because of the crowds at the ultra-famous Cliff Palace. But wait—there's a remedy for that. Show up here when no one else wants to. The crowds at Mesa Verde are somewhat predictable: folks staying in town don't get to the ruins before 9am, school buses aren't here until after 9am, and the earliest tours don't start until 9am. So when do you want to be here? How about BEFORE 9am. We suggest you stay in the park—it's really quite a beautiful view despite the recent scorched-earth of the mesa trees—and get up early. All the park roads are open by 7am. You can have Cliff Palace and many other special lookouts to yourself if you make a point of going as early as possible. Another good bet is during the week in the off season. The crowds are curtailed and the setting is enhanced because of it.

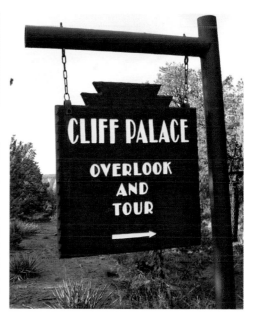

(Artwork by Vernon Morris)

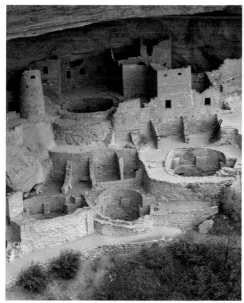

*Tours of Cliff Palace are very popular, so sign up early.*

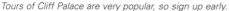

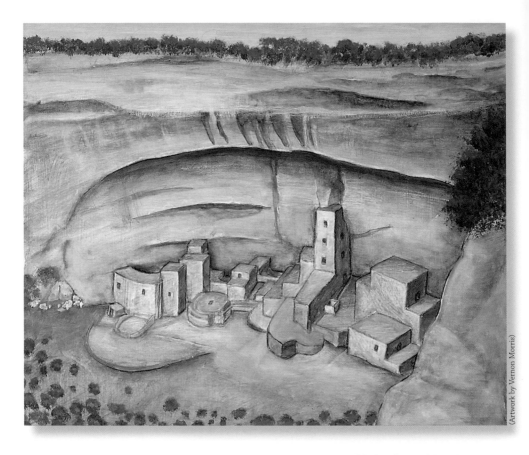

(Artwork by Vernon Morris)

*Square Tower House Then (above) and now (right).*

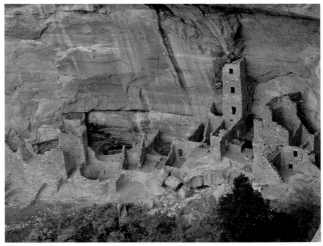

## GET INTO IT

Unlike some monuments where the ruins are off-limits and/or you don't stand a chance at ever getting to them, Mesa Verde is a very interactive experience, with trails running right along and, sometimes even through, ruins, rock art and important sites. One of my favorites is the Petroglyph Trail which starts at Spruce Tree House and winds among the rocks and minor dwellings along the walls as it snakes its way to the canyon entrance. Once there you'll find a fantastic panel of petroglyphs as well as get a great view of the surrounding landscape.

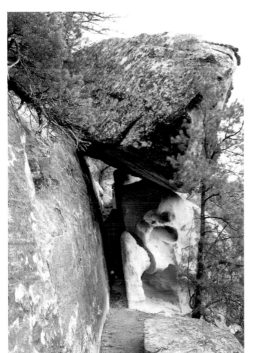 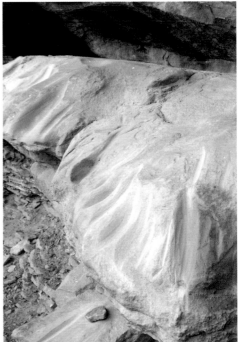

*Believe it or not—the trails are fun and educational as well (left), winding through rock tunnels and (right) passing by strange carved stone slabs along the Petroglyph Trail.*

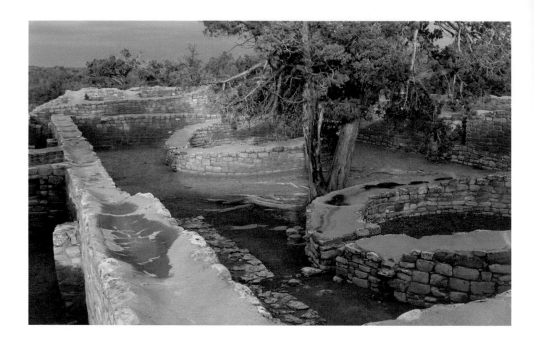

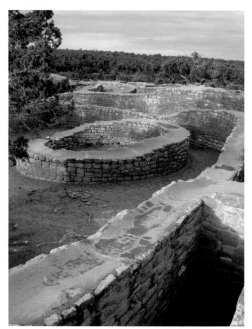

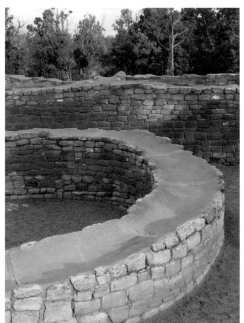

*Sun Temple is just one of the many fantastic ruins which are not tucked away in the nooks and crannies of a cliff overhang. Instead it sits atop the mesa with a commanding view of the canyons below. This, combined with the fact it shows no signs of ever being inhabited, leads to speculation that it may have been a ceremonial structure. It's an enigma to this day.*

## LIVING ON TOP

When imagining Mesa Verde, everyone has the same picture: Huge, elaborate cliff dwellings of multi-story structures rich with artifacts and culture heritage that dominated the landscape as the primary town and religious centers of the entire region. Ironically, most of the area inhabitants probably didn't live in these cliff houses—they occupied great pueblos on the mesa tops (one of which is Far View House, itself home to over 500 inhabitants). Area tenants also lived in community mega-centers in Montezuma Valley, towns whose populations may have dwarfed that of Mesa Verde. It's possible the cliff dwellings were a matter of convenient housing plats, rather than necessary fortifications for the populace.

(Artwork by Vernon Morris)

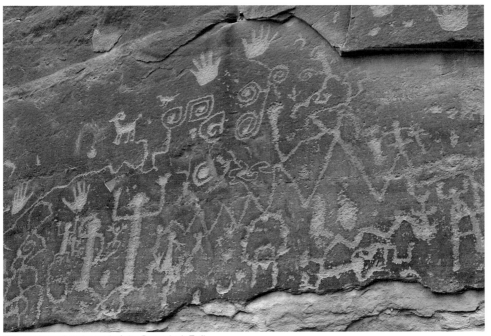

*The cool panel at the end of the Petroglyph Trail.*

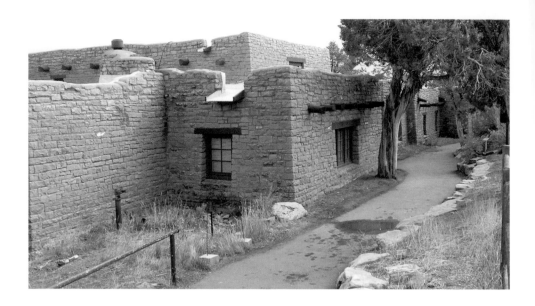

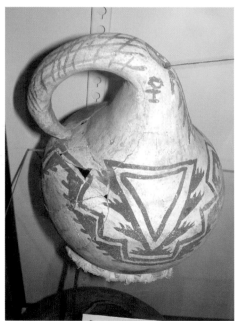

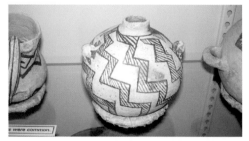

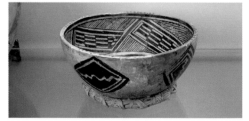

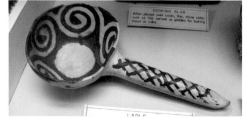

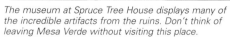

*The museum at Spruce Tree House displays many of the incredible artifacts from the ruins. Don't think of leaving Mesa Verde without visiting this place.*

## NOT MUCH VERDE

Mesa Verde is not a very verde mesa these days. Five consecutive years of fires have swept the mesa since 2000, razing much of the trees in the park. Eerie, charred black forests now stand sentinel along the mesa tops, landscapes whose once-verdant trees gave the park its name. Fortunately, there was little to no impact on the ruins for which this place is famous. On the bright side, the future growth will be more green and lush than ever and in a few years it will be hardly noticeable.

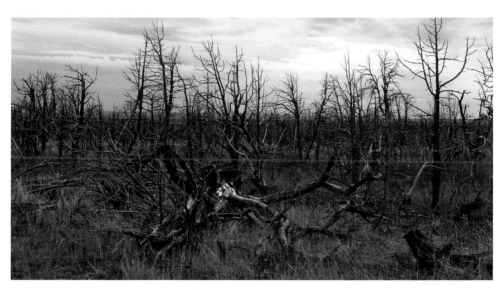

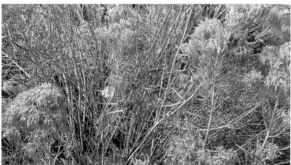
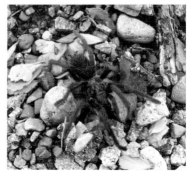

*Fires are, and have always been, a natural part of this environment. They bring nourishment into the soils and provide for new growth. Eventually Mesa Verde will be more "verde" than ever.*

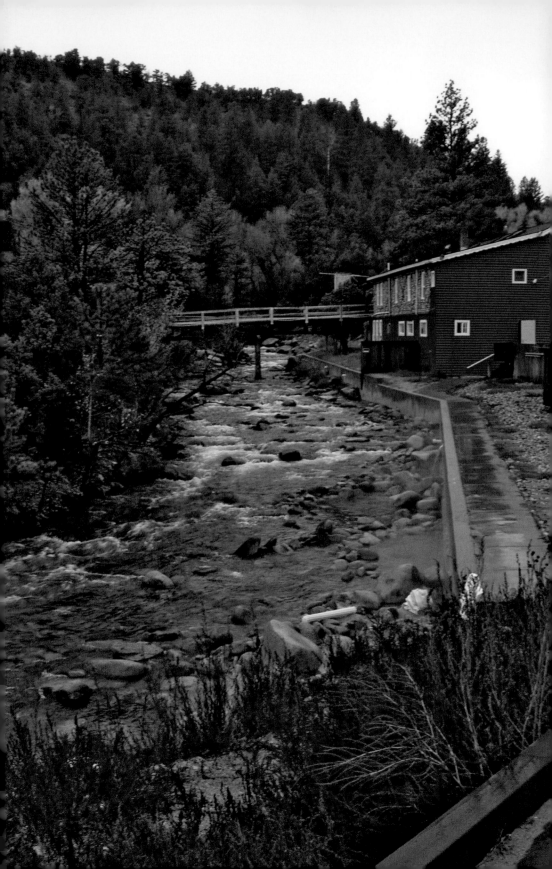

# MT. PRINCETON HOT SPRINGS

**Directions:** From Salida head north on CO 291 and then north on US 285 for a total of about 17 miles. Just before Nathrop, turn west on county 162 toward St. Elmo (patron saint of what?). The resort is 4²/₅ miles just after the bridge.

**Contact Info:**
Mt. Princeton Hot Springs Resort
888-395-7799
www.mtprinceton.com

**Fee:** per person entrance fee

**Hours:** springs and pools access hours vary by season

**Best time to visit:** when it's cold and rainy, a soak in the nice warm springs will reinvigorate you

**Camping/Lodging:** camping nearby; quality lodging on-site

**Access:** easier, cleaner and more fun than most hot springs adventures

**Jon's Rating:** ★★★☆☆ (geology)

**Jon's Notes:**
Hot spring resorts in Colorado are like Christmas Shops at the North Pole—they're everywhere. The problem with most of them is they've destroyed the original natural springs long ago and are piping the thermal waters into prefab baths, spas, and pools. And, yes, the same thing happens here as well. However, there are two very redeeming factors at Mt. Princeton Hot Springs—some natural "hot spots" still occur in the river (just as they always have) and, due to its very low mineral content, the water here is some of the cleanest you'll find anywhere. Unlike many other hot springs, this one doesn't feel greasy and it doesn't smell of rotten eggs.

*LEFT: It's not like it used to be when the Utes had it, but it still has a nice natural setting.*

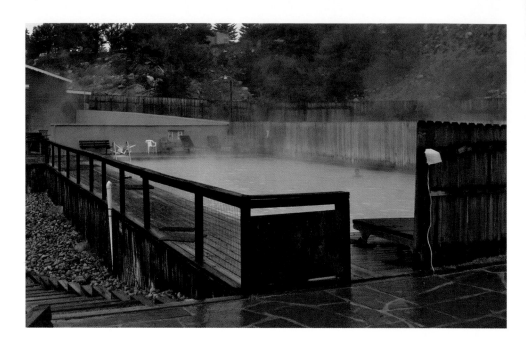

*The setting is the same as it's always been and the water is among the most pure of all Colorado hot springs.*

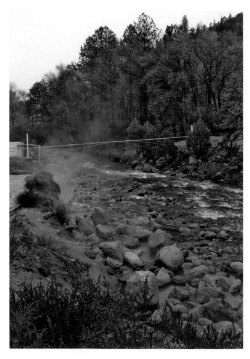

## UTE SCOOT BOOGIE

Originally, the hot springs, which flowed from several vents along the banks of Chalk River, were utilized by local Ute tribes. In the mid-1800s a government surveyor, D.H. Heywood, laid claim to the springs and was granted same despite the fact the Utes had title to the land through a treaty. Heywood developed a resort around the springs he'd finagled from the Utes and built the stone and timber bath house which is still used today. Fortunes of the various resort owners rose and fell with the area mining. Today it is a tourism-based industry which appears more stable financially, if recent development and expansion are any indication.

*You can choose between the big pool or the natural "hot spots" along the river.*

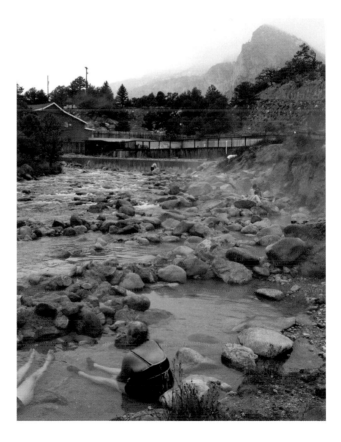

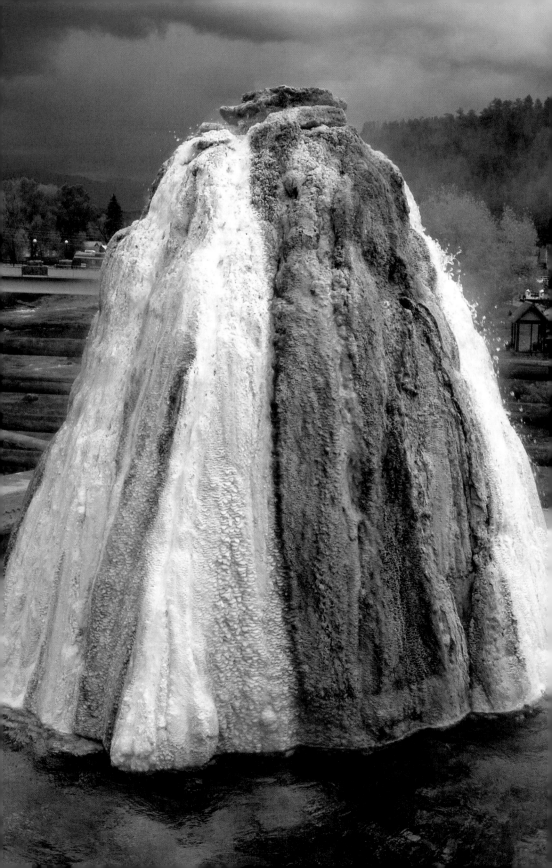

# PAGOSA SPRINGS

## 28

**Directions:** Pagosa Hot Springs is in Pagosa Springs—imagine that. The original hot springs pool—not open to bathing—is behind the main resort complex on the west side of the San Juan River. The bathing pools and tubs are along the river and only accessible from the resort, which charges a fee, naturally.

**Contact Info:**
Pagosa Springs Chamber of Commerce
800-252-2204
www.pagosaspringschamber.com

**Fee:** per person entrance fee for the hot pools, but you can walk around and see the original hot spring and all the neat mineralization sculptures free

**Hours:** access is year-round extended hours

**Best time to visit:** in the rain or snow

**Camping/Lodging:** improved camping and lodging in town

**Access:** easy—just jump in (after paying, of course)

**Jon's Rating:** ★★★☆☆ (geology)

**Jon's Notes:**
There's just no other place in the state which has such active and colorful geothermal mineralization (mineral growth) as Pagosa Springs. The hot springs here are so mineral-laden they form multicolored growths reminiscent of cave formations along and over the rocks through which they flow. The city has installed spring outlets along the walking trails where the towers of calcium have evolved into bonafide civic sculptures complete with "Keep Off" signs.

*LEFT: The natural mineralizations that occur at the outflows are colored by various species of bacteria, making this one of the more interesting hot springs.*

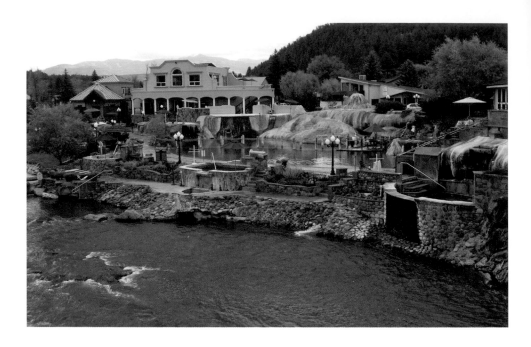

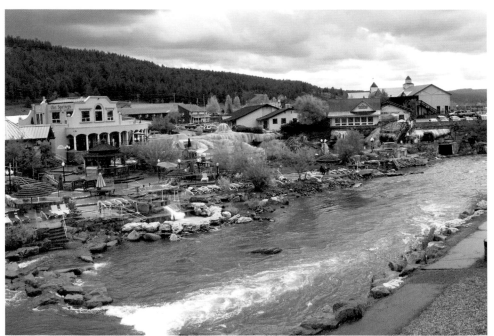

*Located along the cold waters of the San Juan River, Pagosa Springs is yet a small town with lots of charm.*

## HEALING WATERS

Thankfully, the city council has seen fit to preserve the original spring pool, which lies in a field behind the resort complex, fenced off from use. On a cold fall or winter morning, with clouds of mist rising from the surface, it's not hard to imagine the Utes and Navajo enjoying the warm "healing waters" centuries ago. Most of the water now has been diverted (look for the piping under the footbridge over the river) for use in the modern heating plant as well as the spa. In 1980, with a grant from the federal government, the town installed a geothermal system that heats a dozen municipal buildings—including two schools—and still has enough left over to please the spa-goers.

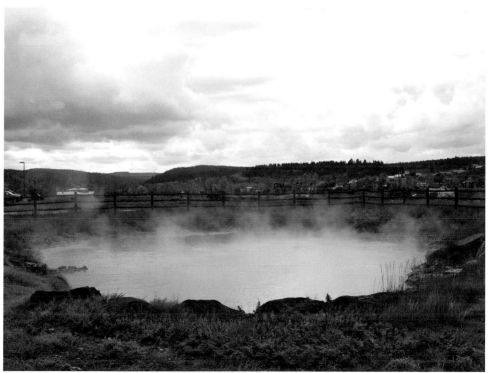

*The healing waters of Pagosa. The original hot springs vent is still preserved behind the resort and you can visit it for free.*

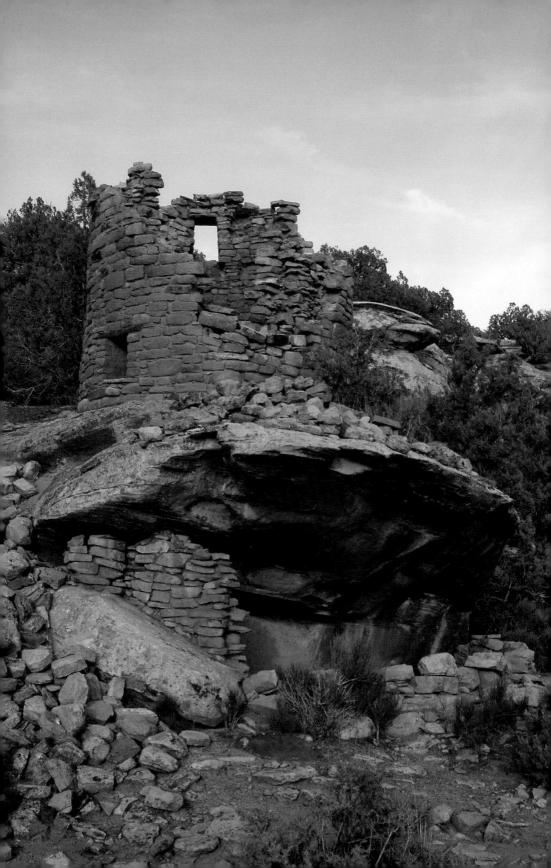

# PAINTED HANDS PUEBLO

## 29

**Directions:** This site is in the center of Canyons of the Ancients National Monument. From Anasazi Heritage Center head west on CO 184 to US 491. Drive north 8.3 miles and turn west on Road BB. Follow for 6 miles to Road 10. Head south for 11³/₁₀ miles. At BLM Rd 4531 turn southeast and drive about one mile to the small parking area overlooking the valley.

**Contact Info:**
Anasazi Heritage Center
970-882-4811
www.co.blm.gov/ahc/hmepge.htm

**Fee:** no fee to see the ruins; museum at heritage center has a modest entrance fee and it's worth it!

**Hours:** year-round daylight hours

**Best time to visit:** whenever the roads are passable, which isn't after a storm

**Camping/Lodging:** basic camping on BLM land for free, but not in, or next to, any ruins; nearest lodging in Cortez

**Access:** the road is paved until you reach BLM 4531; if it's wet or raining do not attempt this road as it becomes a quagmire where you'll be the quag in the mire; once there it's a short moderate hike to the ruins

**Jon's Rating:** ★★★★⯪ (archaeology)

**Jon's Notes:**
In the center of Canyons of the Ancients monument, down a bumpy dirt track, lies a small parking area overlooking a slight canyon and the valley below. When you first look out over the scene you'll say to yourself, "Nice view, but where are the ruins?" Eventually, to the left, you'll notice a fallen wall here, an eroding tower there, and that's only the beginning. Once you climb down along the canyon walls, the fun really begins, as you find ruins tucked away among the boulders and crevasses. There are dozens upon dozens of sites in the immediate area. Your challenge is to find the time to locate them all. I doubt if anyone ever has.

---

*LEFT: One of the nicest little unexcavated ruins in Canyons of the Ancients National Monument.*

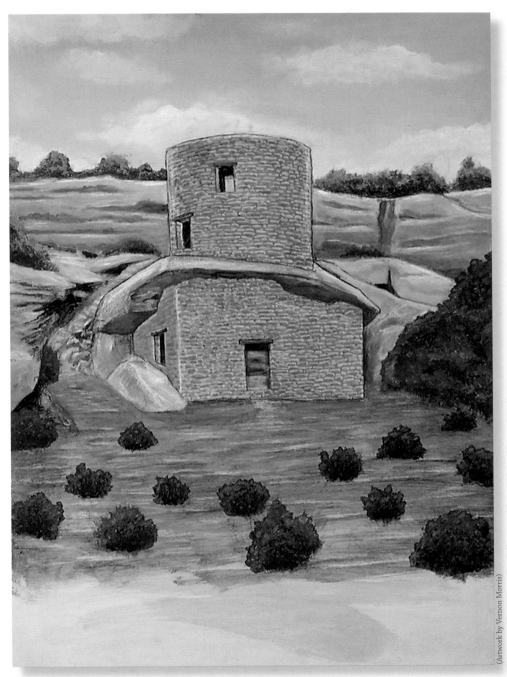

(Artwork by Vernon Morris)

*A condo developer's dream—tower above and storage below. Painted Hands Pueblo, the way it once was.*

## PICTOS AND PETROS

While you're wandering around discovering ruins it may come as a question why someone named this place "Painted Hands Pueblo." The answer lies in a very subtle set of pictographs in the back of a shelter below the prominent round tower. Please do not enter the shelter. Rather, look closely and you will see very faint outlines of hands silhouetted in light bluish hues. At a nearby structure there are petroglyphs but they, too, are nearly hidden. HINT: They are at the base of a sizable right wall on a rock face outside what was once the building.

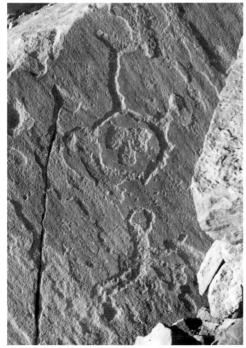

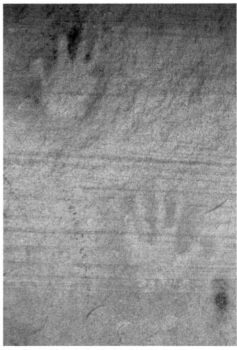

*The rock art here is very subtle and faint. Please do not touch them—not even once.*

*The Painted Hands for which this site is named.*

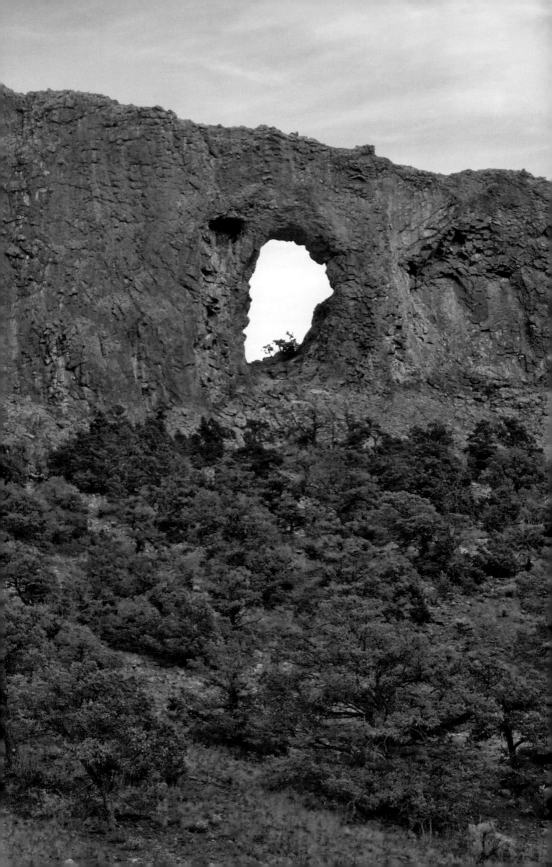

# PENITENTE CANYON & NATURAL ARCH

## 30

**Directions:** To reach the canyon from Del Norte, head northeast on CO 112. In 3 miles turn north onto county 33, which becomes county 38A. After about 9 miles turn left on Penitente Canyon Road. The road ends in about a mile at the parking area. To reach the arch, follow county 38A back south from Penitente Canyon about 3 miles. Turn west on FR 660. In 5$^1$/$_2$ miles turn right on FR 659. Follow 1$^3$/$_5$ miles to the arch, such as it is.

**Contact Info:**
Rio Grande National Forest
719-852-5941
www.fs.fed.us/r2/riogrande

**Fee:** no fee

**Hours:** year-round

**Best time to visit:** don't drive all the way out here on a nice weekend in the summer; you'll find it crowded to the point of not being able to park; rather, visit sometime during the week or, better yet, in the spring or fall

**Camping/Lodging:** basic camping at Penitente Canyon; nearest lodging in Del Norte

**Access:** easy–moderate; it can also get extreme if you're in the mood for rock climbing; the routes here go up to 5.12c

**Jon's Rating:** ★★★✫☆ (geology)

**Jon's Notes:**
One man's Hole-in-the-Wall is another man's Natural Arch. Such is the case here where a vertical slab of rock—actually an igneous dike—has developed a sizeable, if not very impressive, hole in it. If you've ever seen the arches of Arizona and Utah you'll be completely under-whelmed by this one and if this was all the area had to offer we'd not even put it in the guide. That, happily, is not the case and a trip to Penitente Canyon will convince you the land here has some truly redeeming characteristics.

*LEFT: Not much of an "arch" by our standards, but when it's all you've got, then you go with it.*

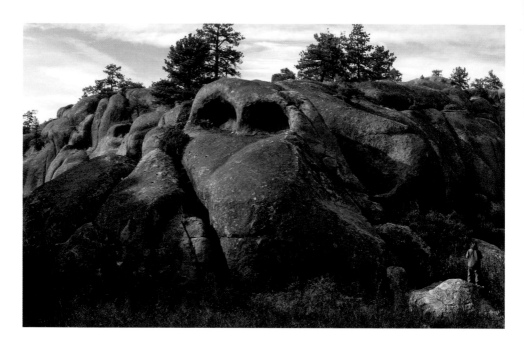

Some very strange rocks abide in Penitente Canyon. Researchers speculate that space aliens may have used this area as a training ground for carving giant stone monoliths. Later, of course, they moved their operations to Mars where they created the giant Elvis statue we've all heard about. American labor unions were pretty peeved about that.

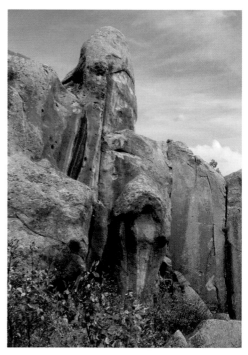

## WEIRD ROCKS

Penitente Canyon is a great little hideaway that you'd never guess was there. Its weird sculpted rock walls form goblin-like figures lining the tiny canyon along which runs an old fault line. It's a natural playground where the kid inside just screams out to climb the wild formations surrounding you. The area has always been a destination for climbers but with a recent surge in magazine and video stories it's become ultra famous in the vertical world. On any given decent-weather weekend the tiny parking lot can be overflowing while the nearby camping area is jam-packed. The resultant scenario is sometimes not very pretty but a hike through the magic canyon is worth every bit of hassle getting to it. If you come on a weekday during the school year you'll likely be rewarded with an easy drive right up to the canyon entrance.

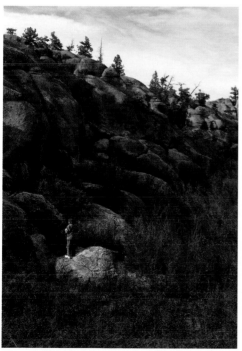

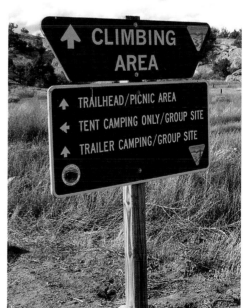

*It's a small and strange canyon but climbers love it.*

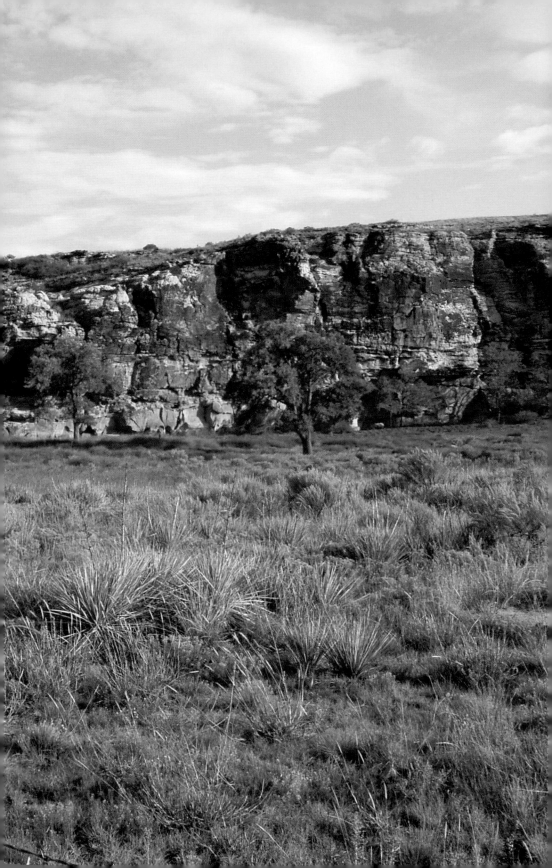

# PICTURE CANYON PICNIC AREA

## 31

**Directions:** From Springfield travel south on US 287/385 about 20 miles to Campo. Turn west on County J. In about 10 miles turn south on County Road 18 and follow the signs to the picnic area, which is about 5 miles farther.

**Contact Info:**
Comanche National Grassland
719-553-1400
www.fs.fed.us/r2/psicc/recreation/camping/coma_picture_picnic.shtml

**Fee:** no fee

**Hours:** daylight hours

**Best time to visit:** anytime the weather permits; spring and fall are especially nice

**Camping/Lodging:** basic camping allowed at the trailhead only, not in the canyon; nearest lodging is in Springfield

**Access:** easy–moderate hiking along maintained trails; watch for snakes in the summer

**Jon's Rating:** ★★★✦✩ (archaeology)

**Jon's Notes:**
Picture Canyon isn't named as such because it's a great place for a photo op. It's the rock art that originally lined its walls that inspired the name. The outstanding "picture" of Picture Canyon is the horse glyph. The horse isn't just a petroglyph, it's also a pictograph, having been colorized after being carved into the sandstone wall. It is located about chest high a little to the right of the first cave you come to. Crack Cave, which is across the canyon, located near the old homestead ruins, is quite possibly an archaeo-astronomy site. During the spring and fall equinox, light penetrates the cavity to a point where certain petroglyphs are illuminated in a special way. This suggests the ancients planned it that way.
The entrance is gated, so you'll have to contact the Forest Service for tours. Contact the Springfield office at 719-523-6591 for a schedule.

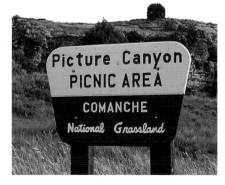

*LEFT: It's a nice place to take pictures of "pictures."*

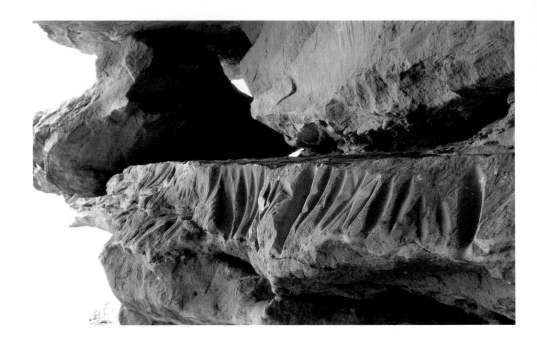

*ABOVE: The caves in Picture Canyon hold interesting things such as these weird grind marks.*

*RIGHT: If you want to see Crack Cave you'll have to call and join a tour.*

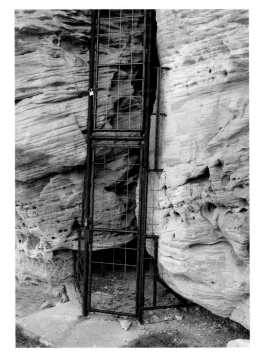

## PICTURE CANYON DREAM

Imagine you're in a dream land of countless centuries ago, a small secluded canyon in a picture-perfect setting, tribes of beautiful native people living in harmony with nature. You float along ethereally through spring-fed meadows rimmed by pastel-colored sandstone cliffs. Native artisans scribe magic symbols along idyllic canyon walls. Slowly you glide up-close to the rock art. As you do you . . . wake up! It was all just a dream and now the reality sets in: the vast majority of the symbols and figures hacked into the rock here are actually the result of 20th

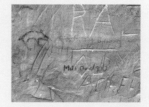

Century lame-brained idiots whose ego got the better of them. It's truly astounding the huge amount of defacement and corruption of the original art. I mean, where did all these people come from anyway? It's hard to imagine a worse collection of graffiti, even if the site was located in Harlem or south LA.

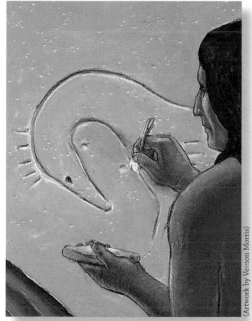

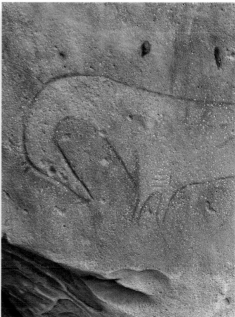

(Artwork by Vernon Morris)

*The famous horse rock art of Picture Canyon.*

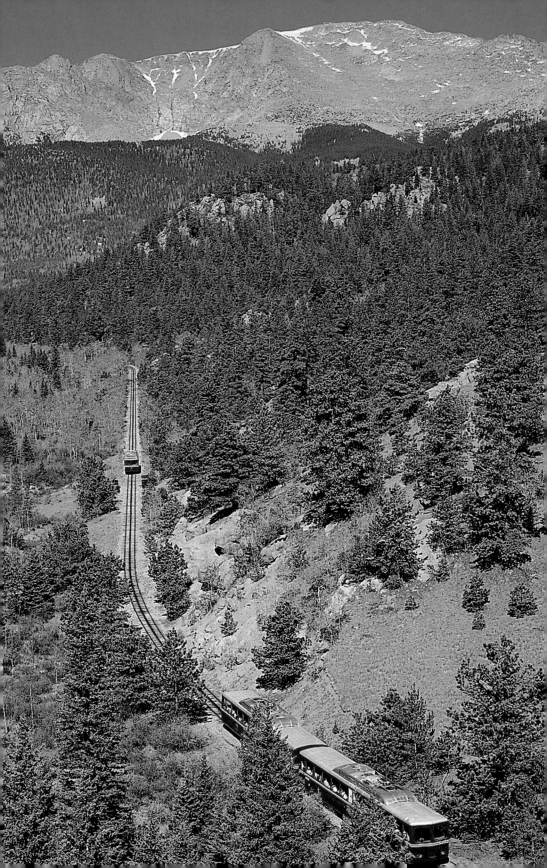

# PIKES PEAK

## 32

**Directions:** You can drive to the top via the North Pole (it's not a joke, it's a tourist trap) or you can save yourself the aggravation of burning brakes and hairpin turns by riding in style via the cog railway. Both start out in Manitou Springs.

**Contact Info:**
Pikes Peak
800-318-9505
www.pikespeakcolorado.com

**Fee:** entrance fee

**Hours:** vary by season and weather—call ahead; surest bet to the top is the cog railway

**Best time to visit:** summer

**Camping/Lodging:** camping and lodging in Manitou Springs and Colorado Springs

**Access:** take your pick from easy to extreme, depending on if you drive, ride the cog railroad, hike, or run in the marathon that goes to the top; the marathon might be a tad difficult

**Jon's Rating:** ★★★½☆ (geology)

**Jon's Notes:**
Although it's undoubtedly the most famous peak in Colorado, Pikes Peak is not the highest (Mt. Elbert, at 14,433' is a couple hundred feet higher). However, it is the most accessible. Unlike the higher peaks, which mostly require vigorous hiking to bag the summit, you can get to the top of this baby in any number of ways—from driving your own vehicle to riding the cog railway. If you're game for something a bit more challenging, why not sign up for the Pikes Peak Marathon (held every August) and go running to the top? You'll be rewarded—if you make it!—at the summit with some hot eats and cool treats at the gift shop/snack bar they cleverly call the Summit House. But you gotta wonder—how did they come up with a name like that?

---

*LEFT: Take the train, take the car, take a hike. You can reach the top in several ways.*

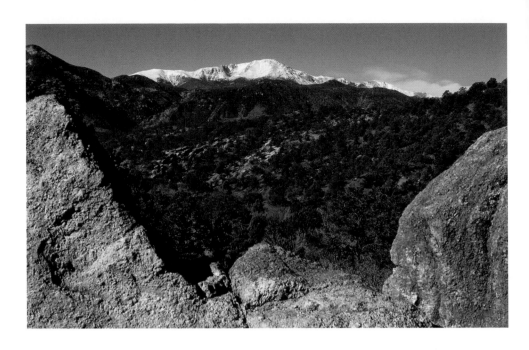

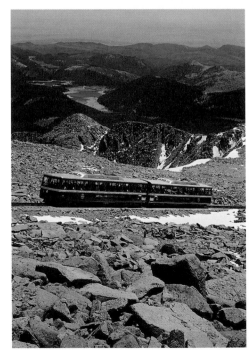

*ABOVE: The peak old Zeb Pike never climbed.*

*RIGHT: When taking the train or driving, pretty soon you find yourself above tree line.*

## ZEB SEZ NO WAY

Zebulon Pike himself would be totally amazed to see how folks are scurrying all over the mountain named for him. Over 500,000 people each year make it to the top! In 1806, when he first saw the peak and attempted to climb it, he was forced to turn back at about 10,000 feet whereupon Ol Zeb declared that the peak might never be climbed! Well, that was then and this is the over-done now, where you can get to the top any number of ways from hiking the Barr Trail, to driving your own car, to hopping a ride on the cog railway. It so happens that this one is the highest cog rails in the world and it has the greatest elevation gain—over 7500 feet. You'll ride in style in heated cars with lots of windows. The line was opened in 1891 with steam engines pushing cars along the track. One of the original iron horses—Engine #4—is kept in good working order, but is used rarely and only for demonstration.

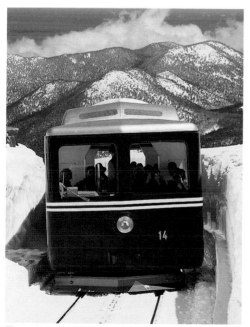
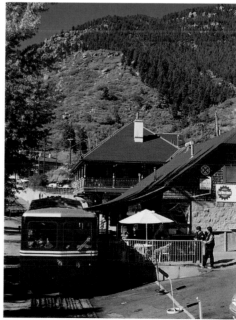

*The train runs anytime it can get through the snow to the top; which isn't every day, especially at times of heavy snowfall in the spring.*

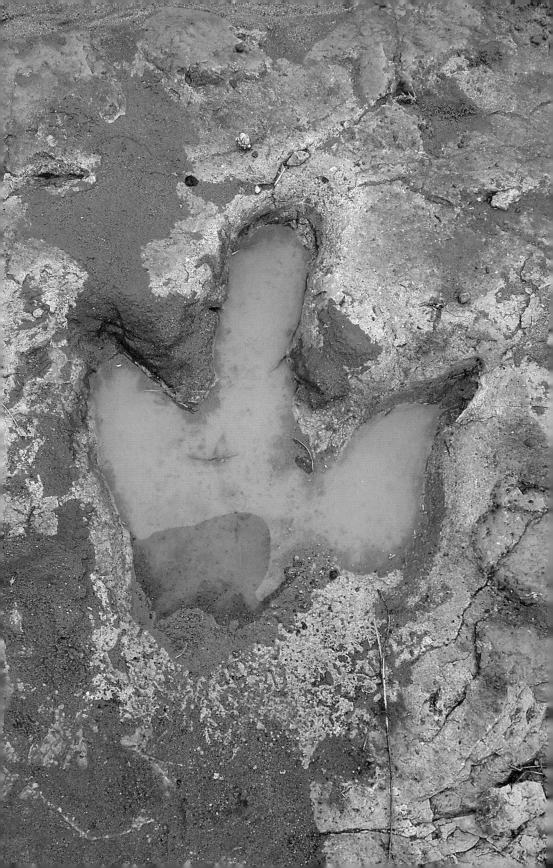

# PURGATOIRE RIVER DINOSAUR TRACKS

## 33

**Directions:** To hike in: From La Junta travel south on CO 109 about 13 miles then southwest on David Canyon Rd for 8 miles. Turn south on Rd 25 (aka Rourke Rd). In 6 miles turn off into the Picketwire Corrals parking area. Take the left gate to Withers Canyon. Follow the main road and signs. In 2 miles bear left at the "T." Follow to end. The hike from here is about 6 miles one-way. OR call the Forest Service for an auto tour of Picketwire Canyonlands and drive right to the dinosaur tracks.

**Contact Info:**
Comanche National Grassland
719-384-2181
www.fs.fed.us/r2/psicc/coma/palo

**Fee:** no fee to enter by foot, however, we highly recommend you sign up for the inexpensive auto tour with USFS

**Hours:** open year-round; auto tours are generally offered on weekends in spring and fall; check the website

**Best time to visit:** avoid mid-summer heat; I like the spring.

**Camping/Lodging:** basic camping at trailhead; NOTE: there is no camping allowed in Picketwire Canyonlands; nearest lodging in La Junta

**Access:** easy–moderate short hike if you take the Forest Service auto tour—it's a moderate 6 miles one-way if you hike in from the trailhead; be sure to carry sufficient water

**Jon's Rating:** ★★★✦☆ (paleontology)

**Jon's Notes:**
Yes, it's Purgatoire alright, but not THAT kind of Purgatoire. Remember those National Geographic stories about the great dinosaurs and how scientists were learning anew about their habits from preserved footprints? Many of the pictures which accompanied the articles were from here. As it happens this is one of the largest dinosaur footprint pavements in the country and many of the impressions show excellent detail.

*LEFT: Is it really Purgatoire or just a long hike in the rain?*

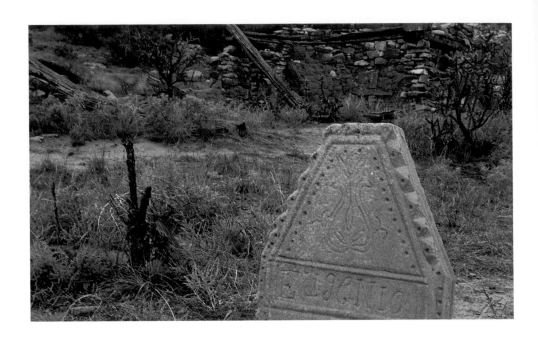

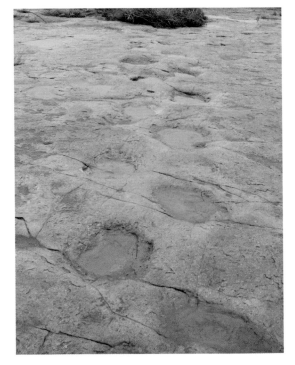

*ABOVE: Some pioneer homesteaders died here in the 19th Century. Hopefully they've worked their way out of Purgatoire by now.*

*RIGHT: WWF championship mud wrestling matches took place here 150 million years ago. Many of the big contenders left their mark.*

## MESOZOIC DINER

As the sign says, many of these tracks could well be "contemporary" with one another, having been stomped into the soft mud about the same time. There's even speculation—based on the trackways in evidence here—that some crafty carnivores were in hot pursuit of a full-meal-deal, chasing a big, juicy T-bone-laden sauropod, across the mud flats. Of course, we don't know if they ever got served, or went hungry that day. Still, if they did, it begs the question—did they get fries with that?

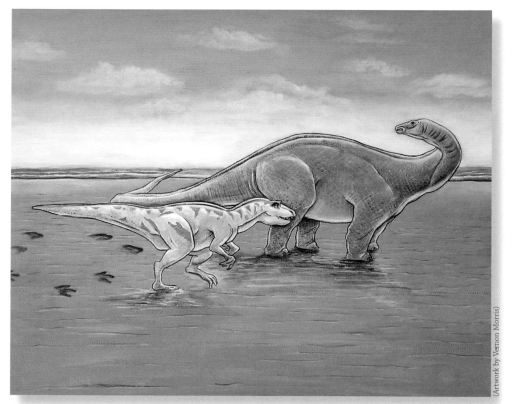

(Artwork by Vernon Morris)

*Shall we dance?*

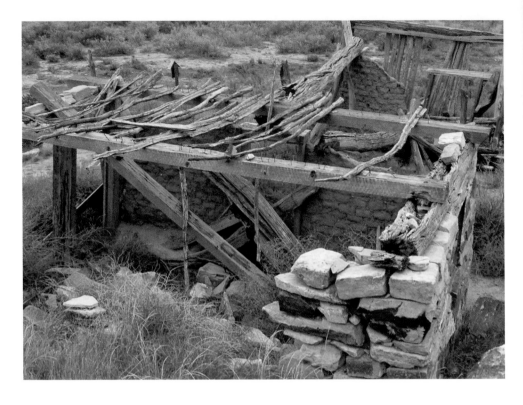

*You'll encounter more than one pioneer homestead along the hike to the dinosaur tracks.*

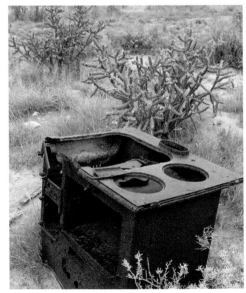

## LOST SOULS

Although the dinosaurs were here first, it was the Spanish that took credit for finding the area. According to legend, in the 18th Century some not-so-lucky treasure hunters died here without the benefit of an ecclesiastic send-off. Upon hearing this rumor, early Spanish explorers named the river "El Rio de Las Animas Perdidas en Purgatorio" (the River of Souls Lost in Purgatory). This cumbersome phrase was shortened—by mandate of the Federal Paperwork Reduction Act or some such bureaucratic device—to Purgatoire River. Despite the gloomy name, enterprising pioneers figured this was a great place to set up homesteads and shortly after that the church followed them. Today, there are some interesting historic sites yet standing along the river valley.

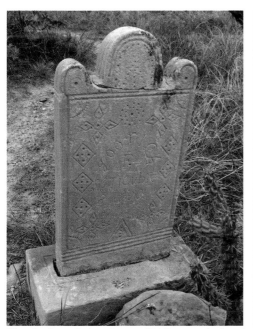 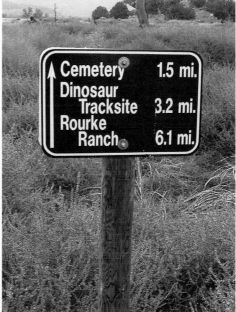

*Signs lead you all along the way (right) so you don't end up like this guy (left).*

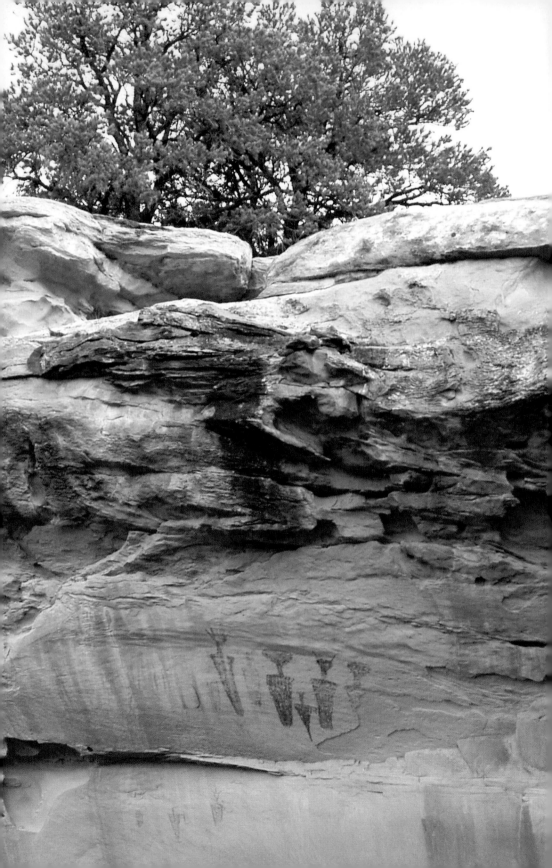

# RANGELY ROCK ART LOOP

## 34

**Directions:** The town of Rangely has developed a clever little tour around the abundant rock art in the immediate area. You can pick up a brochure at the Chamber of Commerce and motels in town. There are over a dozen sites featured with exact directions. Many of the sites are right along CO 139 south of town in the Canyon Pintado Archaeological Area.

**Contact Info:**
Rangely Chamber of Commerce
970-675-5290
rangely.com

**Fee:** no fee

**Hours:** year-round daylight hours

**Best time to visit:** summer and fall

**Camping/Lodging:** basic camping on BLM but not in or next to the sites; nearest lodging is at Rangely

**Access:** most are easy; some are moderate; all are fun; several sites have excellent interpretive signs

**Jon's Rating:** ★★★★☆ (archaeology)
★★★☆☆ (geology)

**Jon's Notes:**
The little town of Rangely was feeling left out: Fruita was cashing in on Colorado National Monument, Dinosaur was cleaning up on dinosaurs, and Estes Park was raking in the dough by showing off a bunch of mountain tops! To add insult to injury even the tiny town of Meeker—located out in the middle of nowhere!—was snagging more than a few travelers with their massacre site. It was a dilemma the Chamber of Commerce decided to meet head on. Unfortunately, try as one might, the idea of a "Rangely National Monument" just wasn't happening. As one local put it, "Heck, all we've got is a bunch of canyons with them darn Indian scrawlings!" BINGO! the idea of the Rangely Rock Art Loop was born.

*LEFT: The area around Rangely is covered with rock art of all kinds.*

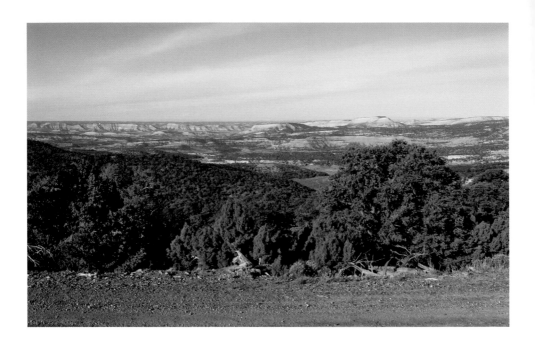

*The settings are spectacular for most of the rock art here.*

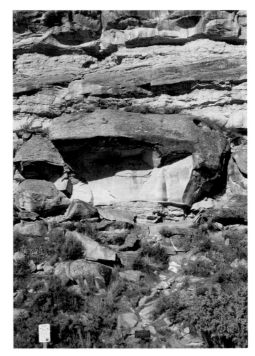

## LOOPY ABOUT ROCK ART

The town Chamber of Commerce has printed a great little brochure describing 16 rock art sites in the area that you can access easily. The trail leads you along a loop south of town, following Dragon Road, through Little Horse Draw and north again along CO 139 back to town. To do the entire loop properly requires a full day or more, although you can just hit a few if you're pressed for time. The brochure has a map and gives exact directions to each location. Pick one up in town at any motel, the Rangely Outdoor Museum, or the Chamber office. I'm not gonna tell you twice that this is a great tour. OK, I will—it's a great tour, now do it!

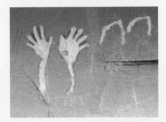

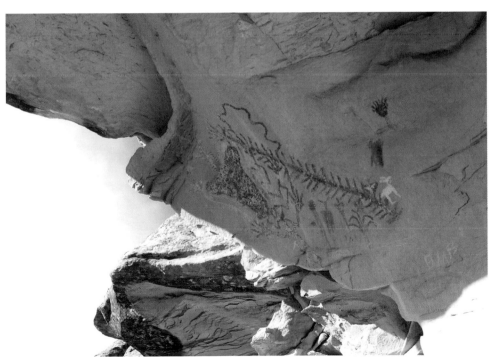

*The art form runs the spectrum from realism to abstract.*

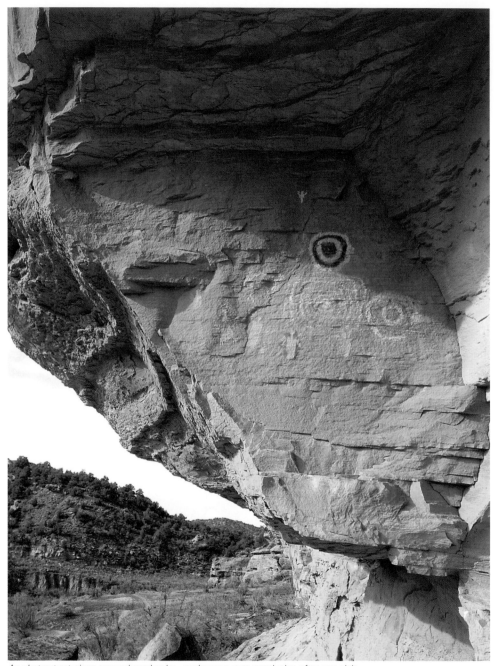

*An abstract art piece or a solar calendar—make your own conclusion after you visit.*

## SUN DAGGERS

It's no coincidence the ancients had "calendars." Ancient Aztecs have had them for millennia. Here there's a site along CO 139 that's important to archaeologists and astronomers, not to mention the ancient farmers who lived here centuries ago. It's listed in the brochure as East Fourmile and is actually a collection of sites along the draw. Of particular interest is the Sun Dagger, a pictograph panel with a display of circles, three of which align along a shadow cast by the sandstone overhang at precisely 10am on June 21—the Summer solstice. There are several other images in the panel, including other circles, but the fact these three line up and are perfectly bisected with the shadow on that date is viewed as more than mere coincidence.

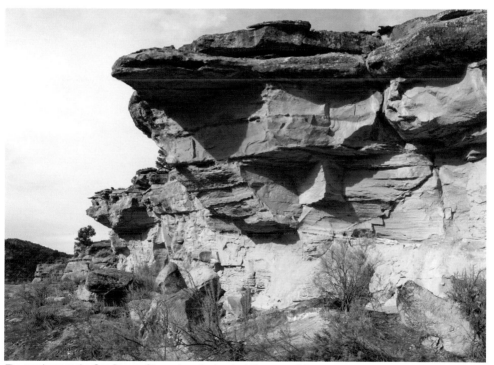

*The overhang at the Sun Dagger Site casts a shadow just like a sun dial.*

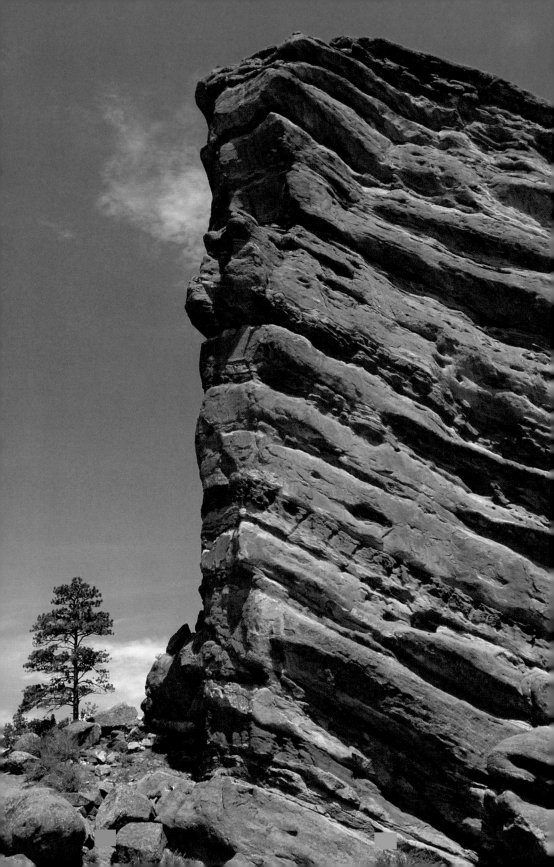

# RED ROCKS PARK & DINOSAUR RIDGE

## 35

**Directions:** From Denver follow I-70 west to exit 259 and head south. In approximately 1 mile or so Red Rocks park entrance will be to your right (west) while the Dinosaur Ridge Interpretive Trail will branch off to your left (east). If you plan it properly you can groove with dinos in the afternoon and party down at a concert that same night.

**Contact Info:**
Red Rocks Park
www.redrocksonline.com
Dinosaur Ridge
303-697-3466
www.dinoridge.org

**Fee:** no fee unless you're at Red Rocks for a concert

**Hours:** the park and ridge are open year-round; hours at the Dinosaur Ridge visitor center are seasonal

**Best time to visit:** when it's a hot day in the city, come on out

**Camping/Lodging:** improved camping and lodging all around but none in the parks

**Access:** you can laugh from the ridge at the rush-hour traffic of CO 470 as you step back in time enjoying the company of dinosaurs; limited parking along the ridge with easy–moderate hiking around these areas.

**Jon's Rating:** ★★★★✦✩ (geology)
★★★✩✩ (paleontology)

**Jon's Notes:**
Back in the good old days when Denver was the center of gold rush mania, it experienced the ups and downs associated with boom and bust of the golden dust. When the Depression hit, the local economy was already in the doldrums and things looked mighty bleak. But then along came FDR and his New Deal to the rescue. The WPA and Civilian Conservation Corps developed plenty of projects around Denver but the Red Rocks park and amphitheater was surely its greatest. The stage and seating areas take advantage of a pre-existing natural depression in the Fountain Formation's 300 million year strata with a view of downtown Denver way off in the distance. The unique acoustics are impressive and, if you ever get a chance to see a concert here, you'll agree there's nothing quite like seeing U-2 rock this park.

*LEFT: Geology is at its finest in Red Rocks Park.*

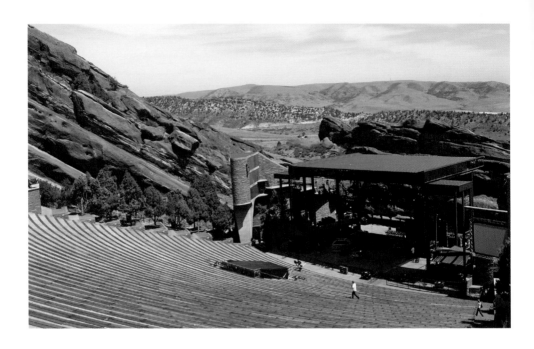

After listening to a heavy-metal rock concert at nearby Red Rocks (above), the leviathans of Dinosaur Ridge left a little tipsy and wandered through some mud holes on their way home (right). Although there were many inebriated individuals, the local police reported no incidents that night.

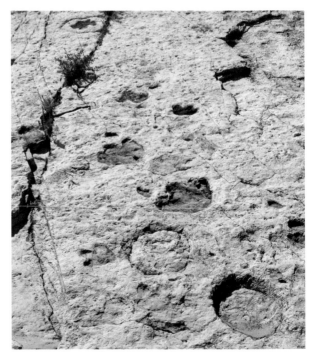

## DINOSAURS ON THE LOOSE

There's nothing quite like seeing the footpaths of fossil animals from eons ago preserved in sediments and revealed to your eyes millions of years later. They tell you things no bones could ever speak. But to see those of several dinosaurs side-by-side and crisscrossing the sediments this way and that, is icing on a very yummy cake. At Dinosaur Ridge you'll have a blast seeing the tracks and, with all the interpretive stations along the route, learning a great deal about the environment that was once this area. Don't forget to stop in at the visitor center at the base of the hill on the east side, there's even more to discover here.

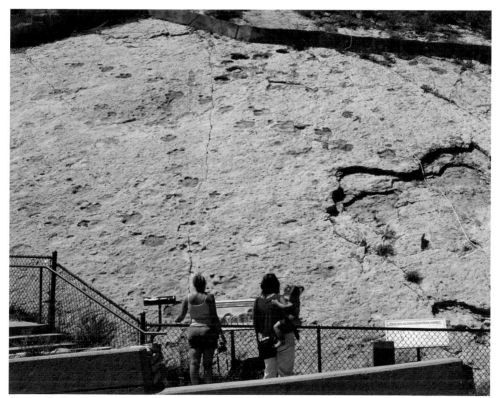

*The excellently preserved dinosaur tracks are right next to the road.*

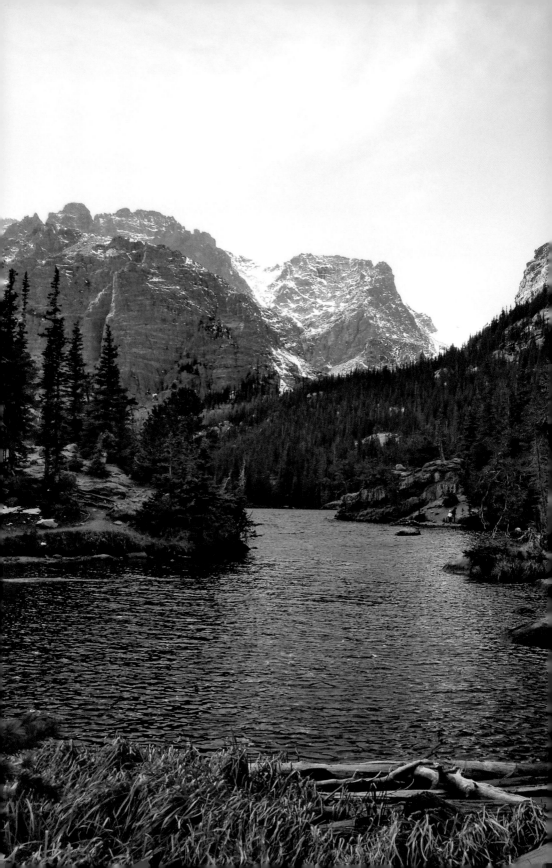

# ROCKY MOUNTAIN NATIONAL PARK

## 36

**Directions:** Go to Estes Park and turn west. If you miss it you have some kind of serious geographic and/or perception problem. You better go get that checked out.

**Contact Info:**
Rocky Mountain National Park
970-586-1206
www.nps.gov/romo

**Fee:** per vehicle entrance fee

**Hours:** park open year-round; road closures and visitor center hours are seasonal and sometimes weather-dependent

**Best time to visit:** summer is always good, but for my money, I'd go for fall—there's less crowds and an easier time getting around the park

**Camping/Lodging:** good variety of improved camping and lodging in the park

**Access:** easy on the drives, moderate–difficult hiking in the back country

**Jon's Rating:** ★★★★☆ (geology)

**Jon's Notes:**
With nearly 400 miles of trail, Rocky Mountain National Park offers endless opportunities to hikers, backpackers, horseback riders, climbers, and just plain car-driving tourists. Anglers, bird-watchers, and photographers have long-since discovered the splendor that these mountains hold and you can too. The park is very "user-friendly" with nice roads and easy access to trails. Elevations range from 8,000 feet in the wet, grassy valleys to 14,259 feet at the wind-swept top of Longs Peak. Processes of glacial geology are a dynamic that still effect the park's personality with an ever-changing environment. Although it's crowded in the "season," the flowerings and wildlife viewing reach their peak in mid-summer.

*LEFT: Come for the view, stay for the peaceful setting.*

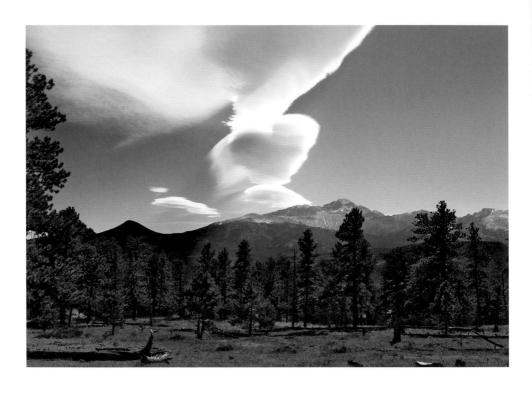

*Seems like every stop
is a photo op . . .*

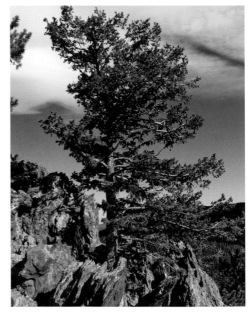

## KEEPING IT NATURAL

When Congress passed the Rocky Mountain National Park Act in 1915, the legislators focused on its scenic and natural wonders. Still, what became the park held many cultural treasures including ancient trails, game drives, cattle ranches, and lodges. Early Superintendents tried to develop roads, back country cabins, and trails to blend with the surroundings. Rangers manipulated the landscape to look more "natural." They suppressed fires, planted seedlings, and controlled predators. During the 1960s, Congress passed significant environmental laws to protect the landscape. Many of these effected the management of both natural and cultural resources in the National Parks. Every year, more cultural resources are identified and protected in Rocky Mountain National Park. Today a team of cultural and natural resource specialists work together to protect the park's resources. The park now hires master carpenters to repair its more than 150 historic structures.

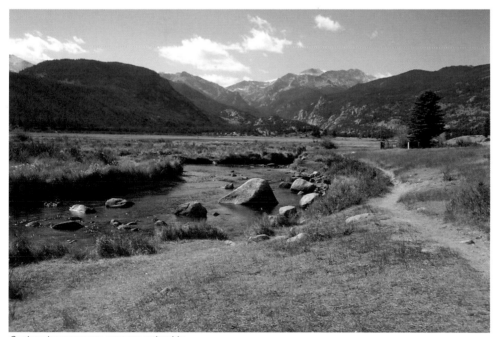

*Geology lessons were never so enjoyable.*

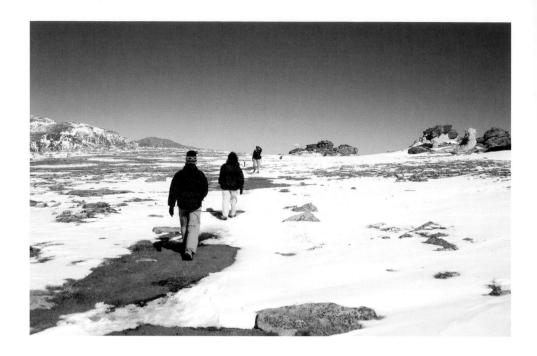

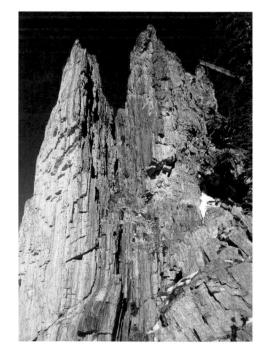

*ABOVE: Mountains? What mountains?*

*RIGHT: Geologic processes are in full vigor here, especially at the higher altitudes.*

## GOLFING WITH THE ELK

So you planned your trip carefully. Being no dummy, you booked it in the fall off-season—less crowds, less cost, more wildlife. Of all the critters large and small you and your family hoped to see it's the elk that every-one was looking forward to. After all, nothing speaks more to the setting here than those bellowing beasts with the huge racks. You've spent the whole week, hiking and driving all over the park but, try as you might, the famous herds have eluded you. The kids are disappointed, your wife is frustrated, and you're at wits end. But it's not your fault—you're not an elk whisperer and the pamphlets all but promised the elk would be here but they're not. There's only one thing to do: Load up the clubs (and kids) and head for the golf course in Estes Park! While you're swinging 18 holes, the family will have its fill of elk watching at the same place. Apparently the municipal golf course is a gathering place for many elk as soon as the weather cools and they come down out of the mountains.

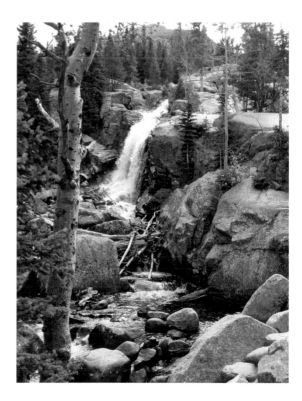

*Travel a little off the road and you can enjoy the peace and quiet of hidden waterfalls in this vast parkland.*

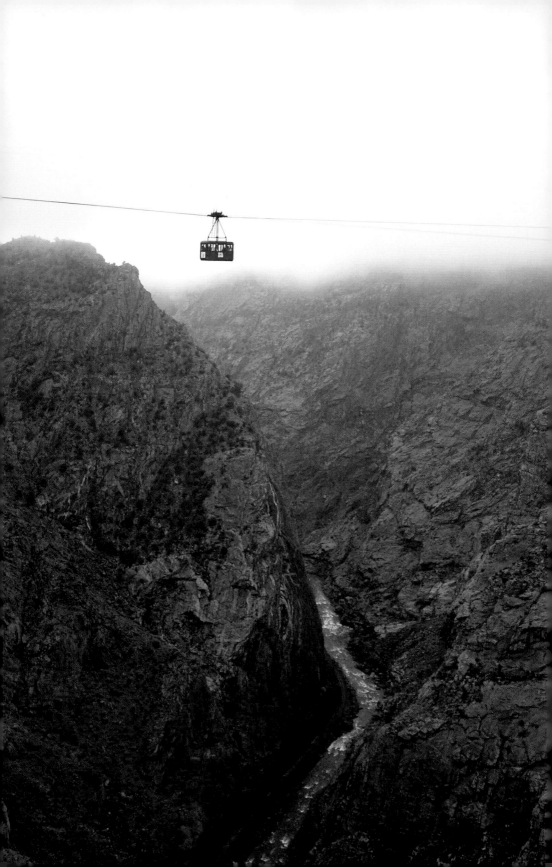

# ROYAL GORGE

**Directions:** From Canon City head west on US 50 about 10 miles to the turnoff at Royal Gorge Junction. Head south and follow the signs.

**Contact Info:**
Royal Gorge Bridge and Park
888-333-5597
www.royalgorgebridge.com

**Fee:** per person entrance fee

**Hours:** hours vary by season—call ahead

**Best time to visit:** summer

**Camping/Lodging:** improved camping and lodging nearby

**Access:** easy and fun, but if you're afraid of heights don't take the gondola ride—opt for the "incline" instead!

**Jon's Rating:** ★★★★☆ (geology)

**Jon's Notes:**
At 1200 feet deep Royal Gorge is one of the deepest canyons of Colorado and certainly the most accessible. The friendly folks at Royal Gorge Bridge and Park have taken the opportunity to help you find your way around by offering every conceivable form of conveyance to experience the Gorge's natural splendor—from walking out on the suspension bridge, to riding the inclined railway to the bottom. You can even take a surreal aerial tram ride across the gaping maw for that extra special feeling. But if you're afraid of heights you may want to opt for a more "terra firma'" experience at one of the many overlooks.

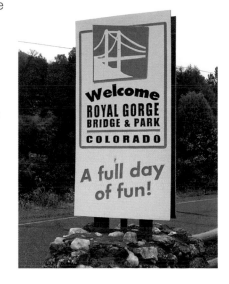

*LEFT: The most royal gorge in Colorado.*

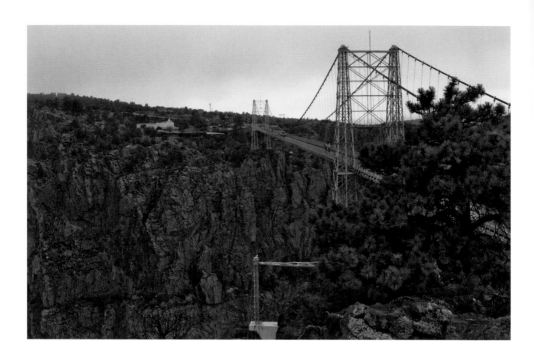

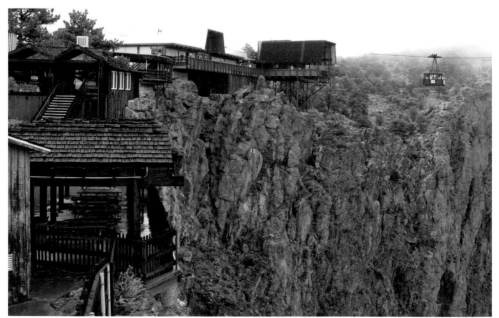

*You can walk or drive across the bridge (top) if you want to do it yourself at your own pace. But for the real adventurer there's the gondola (bottom).*

## THE ROYAL GORGE WAR

In 1877, silver was discovered on the upper waters of the Arkansas River. This sparked a controversy between two competing railroads: the Rio Grande and the Santa Fe. Both wanted the rights to build the new freight railroad to carry the ore down from the mountains. Things got a little hairy as the two sides dynamited each other's rail lines and took pot shots at survey parties. The "Royal Gorge War" eventually evolved into a six-month court battle. The Santa Fe wasn't very happy with the results and decided to press the matter by hiring legendary gun fighter and U.S. Marshal Bat Masterson and his Kansas posse to help protect their crew and materials. The Rio Grande countered with a 200-man posse led by former Governor A.C. Hunt. Might isn't always right, but the Rio Grande railroad eventually won out, both in court and in the gorge.

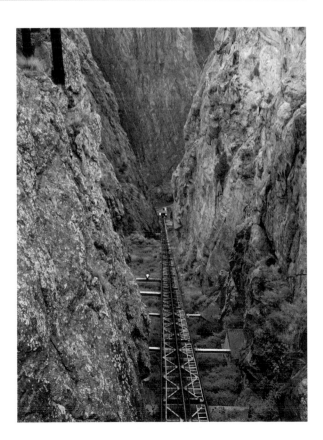

*Now you're talking! It's an inclined railway that takes you to the bottom while allowing you to sip cokes without leaning to one side or standing on your head.*

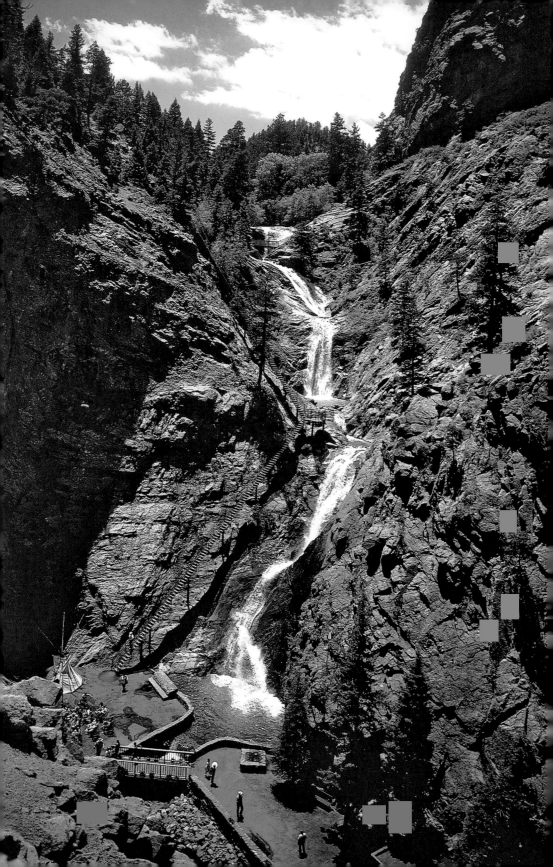

# SEVEN FALLS

**Directions:** From Colorado Springs follow Cheyenne Blvd, west to the falls.

**Contact Info:**
Seven Falls
719-632-0765
www.sevenfalls.com

**Fee:** per person entrance fee

**Hours:** spring/fall 9am–5:15pm; mid-May through Memorial Day 8:30am–9:30pm; June through mid-August 8:30am–10:30pm; winter 9am–4:15pm

**Best time to visit:** summer and fall; for a special treat, visit at night and see the light show

**Camping/Lodging:** camping and lodging in Colorado Springs

**Access:** easy–moderate depending on how rambunctious the kids are and how many times you have to chase them up and down the 224 steps

**Jon's Rating:** ★★★☆☆ (geology)

**Jon's Notes:**
I'm a fan of waterfalls—negative ions move me. And if one waterfall is good then many waterfalls are better, especially if there're several in a row. Yes, some other waterfalls in the state are taller, and others still that have more cascades. But none combine to create a spectacle such as this in a site so easily accessed. Here you have a 224-step walkway adjacent to the falls themselves. If you're not that energetic, you can ride the "in-mountain" elevator to the top. As the sign says, it's been blasted 14 stories straight up through Pikes Peak Granite to

the Eagle's Nest over-look. Rumor has it there have even been Elvis sightings here.

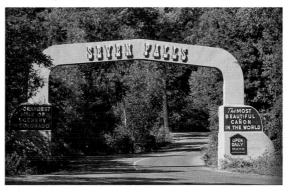

*LEFT: You don't have to climb all the steps—there's an elevator!*

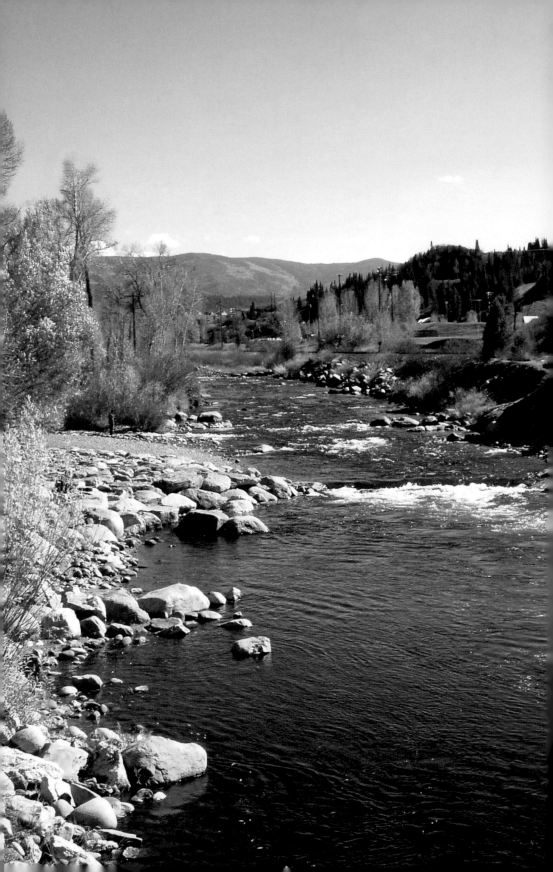

**Directions:** There's a lot of springs in Steamboat Springs but the best learning experience is on the northwest side of town at the springs walking tour which begins at Lincoln and 13th, next to the library.

**Contact Info:**
Steamboat Springs Chamber of Commerce
970-879-3495
www.steamboat-chamber.com

**Fee:** no fee for the walking tour of the springs

**Hours:** anytime you're game, the springs are too!

**Best time to visit:** anytime, even in the dead of winter

**Camping/Lodging:** improved camping and lodging in town

**Access:** easy walk; just be careful around the streams and pools as wet rocks can be very slippery

**Jon's Rating:** ★★★★☆ (geology)

**Jon's Notes:**
There're springs all over this town! Springs that are hot, springs that are cold, and springs that are warm. White springs, black springs, even purple springs. There's springs spewing rust and some belching sulfur. And, for those in need of real medicine, there's even a spring that has lithium in its waters. In short, you will not find another place on Earth that has such a tremendous variety of geothermal springs in such a small area. There are over 150 different springs in Steamboat.

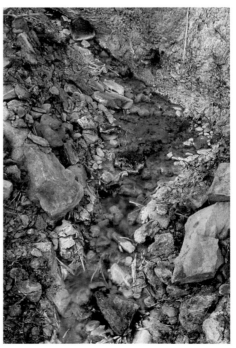

*LEFT: Most of the springs occur along the Yampa River.*

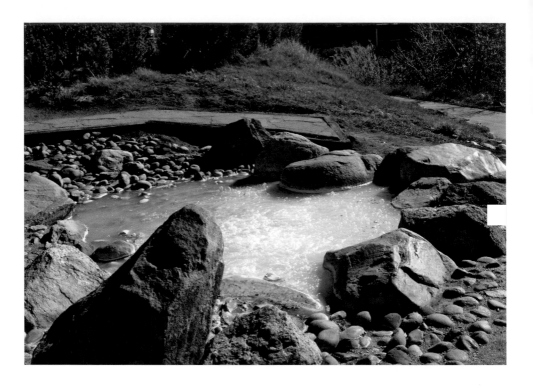

*The sheer variety of springs in town is amazing. Many have interpretive signs.*

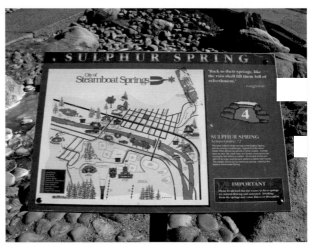

## STEAM YES, BOAT NO

Legend has it that Steamboat Springs was named by some misguided French fur trappers in the 1860s. After losing their bearings and wandering the mountains for several months, they came along a ridge whereupon they heard what they thought was the distant horn of a steamboat along a river. At last! They could hitch a ride to civilization and finally sleep in a cozy bed. Well . . . they got the steam part right, and even the whistle to a degree, but there was not much of a river, and certainly no steamboat. Upon closer examination they found their "steamboat" was actually a hot spring that periodically blasted it's own steam out and happened to whistle while doing it. With this discovery, the trappers were not happy campers, being forced to carry on with their own two feet.

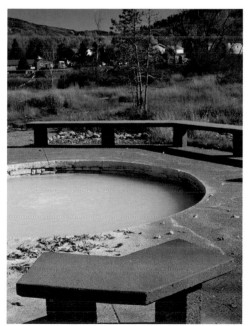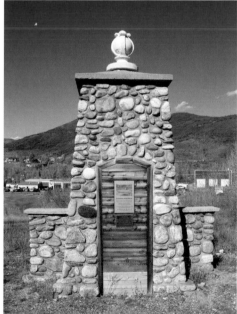

*Some years ago this particular spring became well known for its calming lithium content. No wonder the kooks all come here . . . They even erected a monument to it (right).*

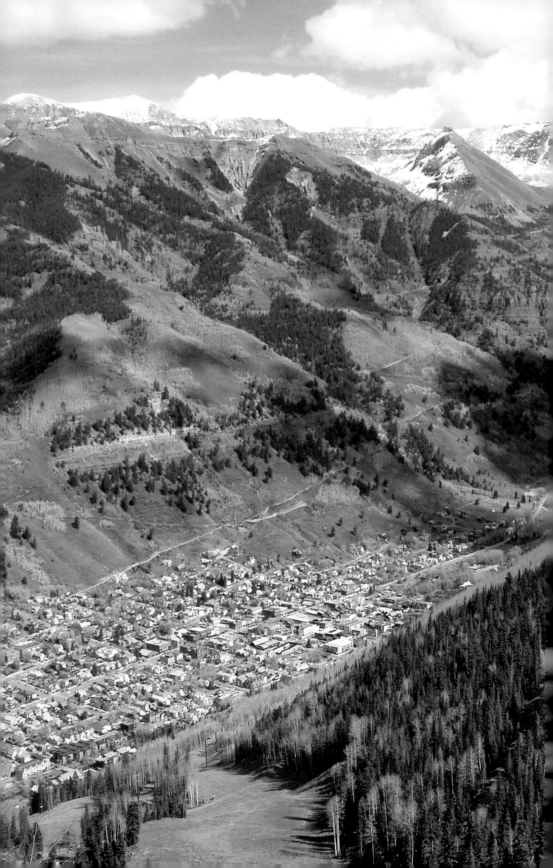

**Directions:** Pay attention here! The only normal driving route into—and consequently out of—Telluride is from the west via CO 145. Don't try and take a shortcut from Ouray, unless you have a jeep and a lot of tolerance for your head banging into the car frame.

**Contact Info:**
Telluride Visitor Information Center
970-728-3041
www.telluridechamber.com

**Fee:** no fee; even the gondola ride is free!

**Hours:** you can get to the falls anytime the weather permits; the free gondola ride from town is open until midnight!

**Best time to visit:** anytime really, but I like it here in the fall best—less crowds and nice colors

**Camping/Lodging:** improved camping and lodging

**Access:** if you come for just the views, then it's all pretty easy; but if you want to get up-close, hiking to the falls is moderate

**Jon's Rating:** ★★★☆☆ (geology)

**Jon's Notes:**
It's in a perfect setting so naturally the place is trendy and upscale. But that's no reason to shun it. The natural scenery here is like something out of Switzerland—high peaks surrounding a nice little valley with waterfalls and cascading creeks. Despite all the development and buildup since the ski resorts opened, the town of Telluride has maintained a sense of old town charm by preserving its historic buildings with strict zoning laws. And the town-supported free gondola ride—year-round!—helps mitigate that $5.00 cup of coffee.

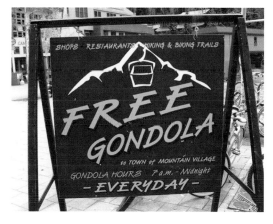

*LEFT: What a setting!*

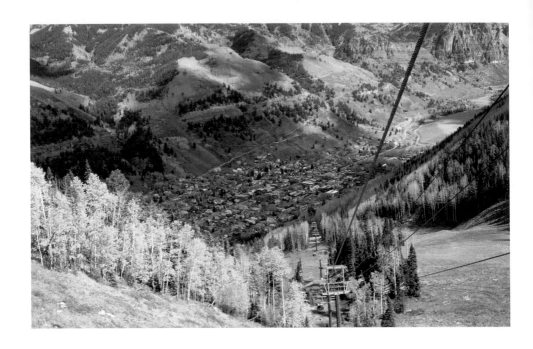

*ABOVE AND RIGHT:*
*There's nothing quite*
*like a view from the*
*top, especially if the*
*ride is free.*

*BELOW RIGHT:*
*There's even a nature*
*center up here.*

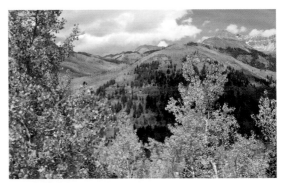

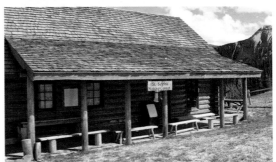

## BRIDES AND FALLS

Why is it people are compelled to name waterfalls after marriage attire? There are dozens of Bridal Veil Falls in the world—there's even one in Yosemite (probably the tallest) and another as part of Niagara Falls (probably the largest). Sure, it's a cute name, but really, can't someone come up with a name that's just a little more creative? How about something futuristic like "Cosmic Veil"? Or a little ecclesiastical as in "Holy Grail Veil"? Oh, what the heck, just leave it, I'll deal with it . . . Whatever you call it, you'll find it by driving through town as far as you can go toward the back of the valley. Bridal Veil Falls plunges over 100' in one drop to the valley floor.

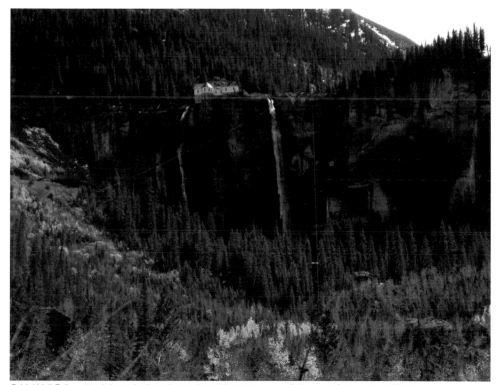

*Bridal Veil Falls—check it out in the winter when it becomes one of the most famous ice pillars in the country.*

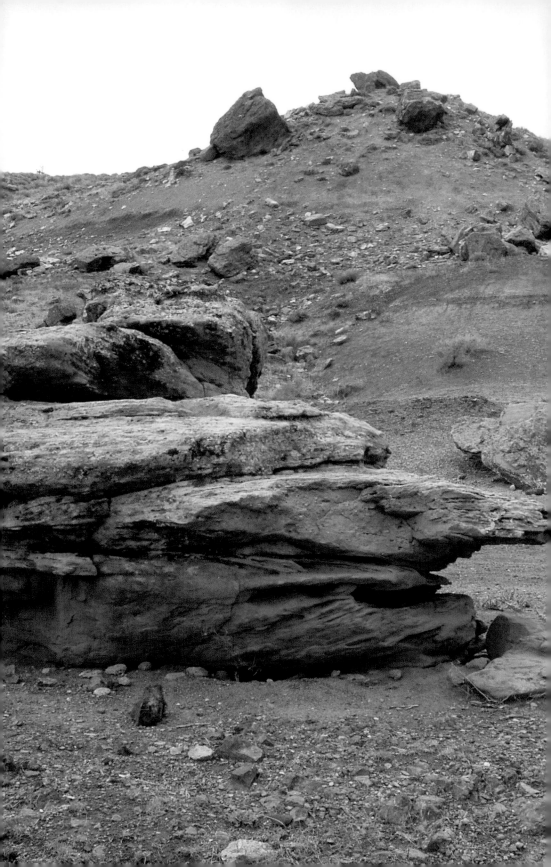

# TRAIL THROUGH TIME

**Directions:** It's not hard to get to. From I-70 take exit #2 and drive north. You will very quickly run out of road and next thing you know you're there! This site is in the newly-designated McInnis Canyon National Conservation Area.

**Contact Info:**
BLM Colorado
970-244-3000
www.dinosaurdiamond.org
www.co.blm.gov/mcnca
www.dinosaurjourney.org

**Fee:** no fee

**Hours:** year-round

**Best time to visit:** spring or fall; avoid the heat of mid-summer

**Camping/Lodging:** basic camping on BLM land in the McInnis Canyon NCA; nearest lodging in Fruita

**Access:** easy or difficult depending on whether you are working at the dinosaur dig in the middle of summer

**Jon's Rating:** ★★☆☆☆ (paleontology)

**Jon's Notes:**
If it wasn't for the signage, there'd not be a whole lot of time travel going on around here. No one would stop, even if they knew about the supposed time warp reported in *Weekly World News*. But there ARE signs and information stations with great graphics and lots of explanations. If you're lucky, you might even stumble upon a research team excavating dinosaur bones out of the hillside while you're here. The spot is known as the Mygatt-Moore Quarry and has yielded several important fossil specimens. Just keep an eye out for Rod Serling from the Twilight Zone—that's when things really get weird.

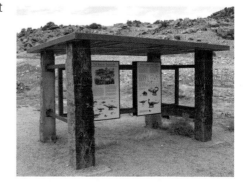

*LEFT: It's a time warp, but at least there's a trail through it . . .*

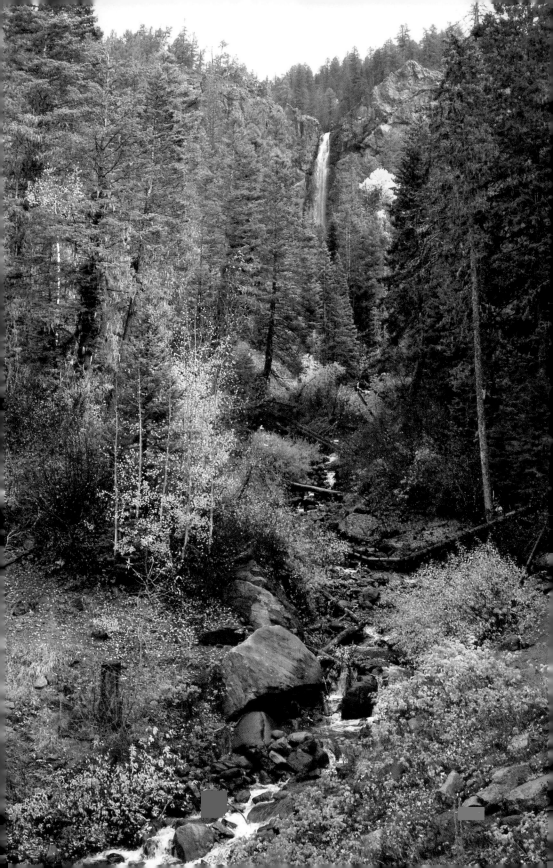

**Directions:** If you are driving west on US 160 from Wolf Creek Pass toward Pagosa Springs, Treasure Falls will be near the bottom, shortly after the main overlook and about the time your brakes will run out of pad.

**Contact Info:**
no visitor center and no phone
www.naturalhighs.net/waterfalls/falls/treasure.htm

**Fee:** no fee

**Hours:** anytime you're driving by

**Best time to visit:** anytime, but the fall colors really bring out the fall's beauty

**Camping/Lodging:** improved camping and lodging in Pagosa Springs

**Access:** easy as it gets—someone conveniently placed Treasure Falls right next to the road

**Jon's Rating:** ★★☆☆☆ (gcology)

**Jon's Notes:**
Even if you're not a big fan of waterfalls, this one is so easy to get to you can't pass it up. If the road was any closer you'd be driving right under it. There is a trail leading to the waterfall's base but the best view is from the road anyway. All you have to do is find the bathroom and you've found the trailhead!

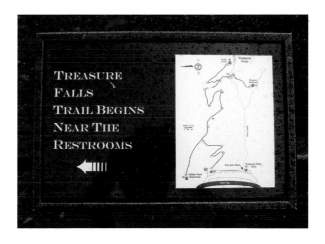

*LEFT: Stop here on your way up from Pagosa Springs or down from Wolf Creek Pass.*

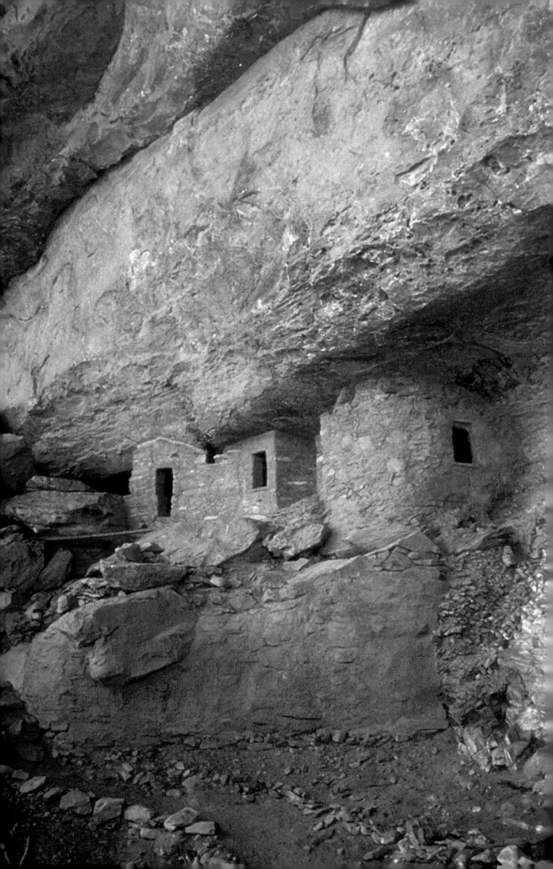

# UTE MOUNTAIN TRIBAL PARK

**Directions:** The Ute Mountain Tribal Park is located 20 miles south of Cortez at the intersection of US 491 and US 160.

**Contact Info:**
Ute Mountain Tribal Park
800-847-5485
www.utemountainute.com/tribalpark.htm

**Fee:** per person fee based on tour type

**Hours:** the ruins are accessed only by reservations, so call at least a day ahead; there are half and full day tours, all of which leave the center at 9am

**Best time to visit:** spring to fall, but make sure it's dry

**Camping/Lodging:** improved camping and lodging in Cortez

**Access:** easy–difficult depending on the sites you visit, the guide you employ, and the route you take; NOTE: if it rains it's a good idea to postpone your adventure

**Jon's Rating:** ★★★★⯪ (archaeology)

**Jon's Notes:**
Although more than twice as large as Mesa Verde, and hosting far more ruins and petroglyphs in a more original state, Ute Mountain Tribal Park is not well-visited. And for you, that's a good thing. Tours are arranged in advance and must be accompanied by a Ute tribal guide. Groups are small, especially in the off-season—sometimes it's only a few people. The trips are from one-half to full-day, using your own car. The experience is unforgettable. Each and every stop has artifacts lying around just as it was found. You therefore get the impression you are one of the very first people to see these incredible sites. It's a genuine archaeological and cultural experience unlike any other.

*LEFT: One of the most authentic ruins tour you'll make.*

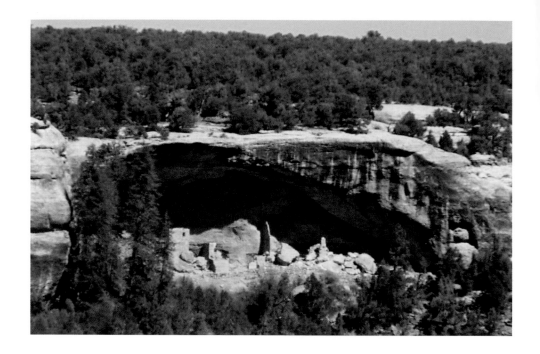

*The ruins at Ute Mountain Tribal Park are much like those found at Mesa Verde, multi-story buildings tucked away in sandstone alcoves. The difference is most of these have never been excavated and are just as they were when first recorded by white survey parties.*

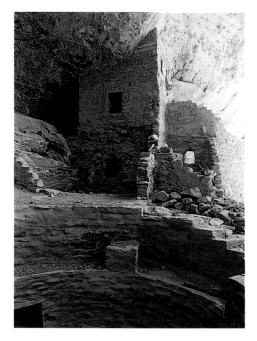

## THE REAL THING

In many ways Ute Mountain Tribal Park is an alternative reality to the Mesa Verde experience. At Mesa Verde many of the ruins have been excavated and stabilized, the crowds can be oppressively huge, and your guide is more likely to be white than any other color. At Ute Mountain, the ruins are just as they have always been (unexcavated), there are no crowds (ever), and your guide is Ute (native). This adds up to a far more genuine archaeological adventure worth every cent of the tour price. Here you'll feel more like Indiana Jones than Inspector Clouseau.

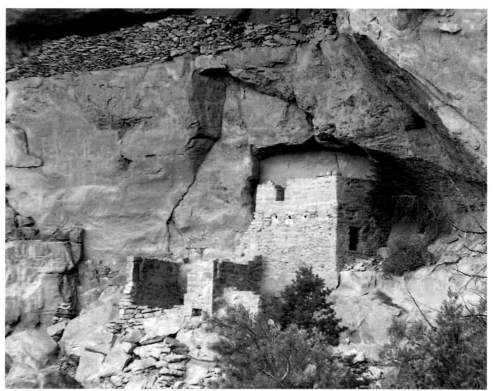

*To see some of the ruins requires a bit of hiking and scrambling, but it's well worth it!*

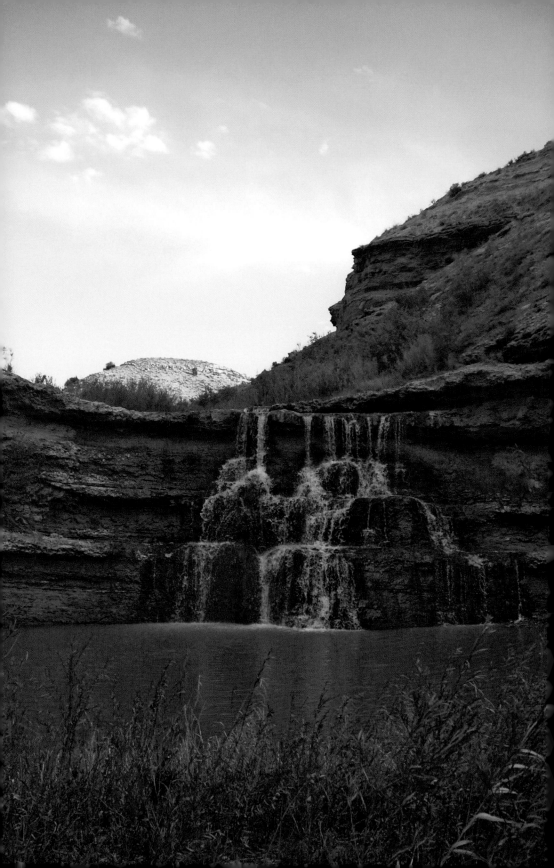

**Directions:** On CO 318 look for mile marker 20. Turn west and keep to the right on the dirt track. This will lead you to the falls in about 1/3 mile.

**Contact Info:** no visitor center, no phone, no website, no nothing!

**Fee:** no fee

**Hours:** year-round

**Best time to visit:** when water is flowing over it—especially in the spring

**Camping/Lodging:** camping at Gates of Lodore or Irish Canyon; nearest lodging is in Craig

**Access:** easy—but don't try it in wet weather—you'll get stuck in the muck and get all mucked up

**Jon's Rating:** ★★★★★ (geology)

**Jon's Notes:**
OK, so it's not a whole lot in the way of falls, but it's a nice stop on the way south from the Gates of Lodore and Irish Canyon. You'll see the falls on the right as you head south. After turning off the pavement, head to the right, down the hill and you'll end up at their base. But do NOT try this in wet weather. The dirt road becomes a quagmire and it's a long, long way back to town.

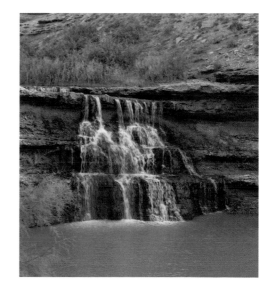

*LEFT: Hey, it ain't much but it's all we have 'round these parts!*

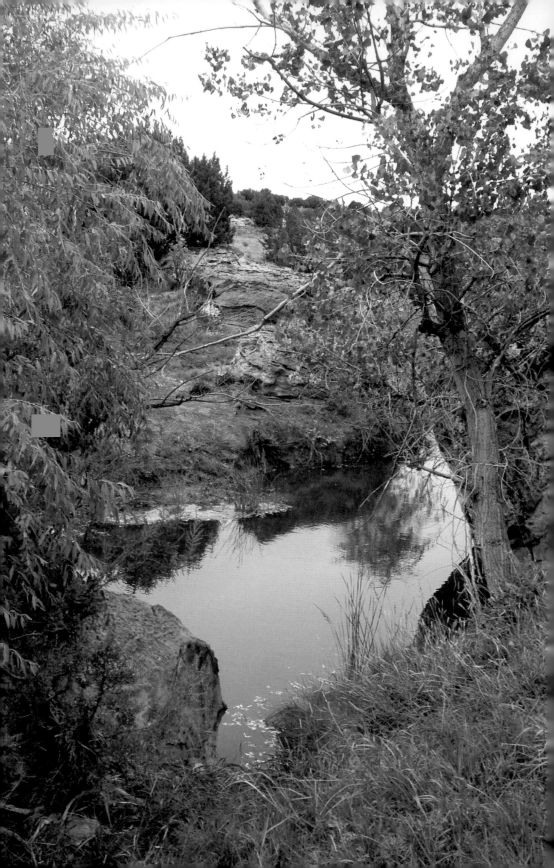

# VOGEL CANYON

## 45

**Directions:** From La Junta travel south on CO 109 about 13 miles, then southwest on David Canyon Rd for 1¹/₅ miles. Turn south and follow main road for 1²/₅ miles to picnic area.

**Contact Info:**
Comanche National Grassland
719-553-1400
www.fs.fed.us/r2/psicc/recreation/camping/coma_vogel_picnic.shtml

**Fee:** no fee

**Hours:** daylight hours

**Best time to visit:** summer and fall

**Camping/Lodging:** basic camping allowed at the trailhead only, not in the canyon; nearest lodging is in La Junta

**Access:** easy–moderate; if the cows are agitated it can get pretty dicey

**Jon's Rating:** ★★★½☆ (archaeology)

**Jon's Notes:**
One of the nice things about Vogel Canyon is there's no guesswork. You know what's expected of you (or rather you're told what's expected of you) and you learn the "who-what-when-where-why" of the canyon inhabitants from the earliest (hunters and gatherers, BC 5500) to the most recent (you, the present). This well-maintained-almost-groomed-site has something to say about most everything, with judiciously posted information stations all along the way. The most conspicuous archaeo-logical features are the rock art panels on the lower walls of the canyon. They are well-marked and interesting, albeit not in very good shape and not all that abundant.

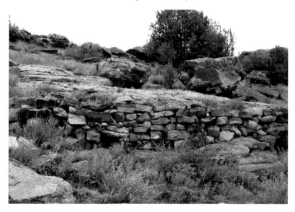

*LEFT: The ancients lived here because this was their water source. That and the fact the parking lots had already filled up over at Wal-Mart.*

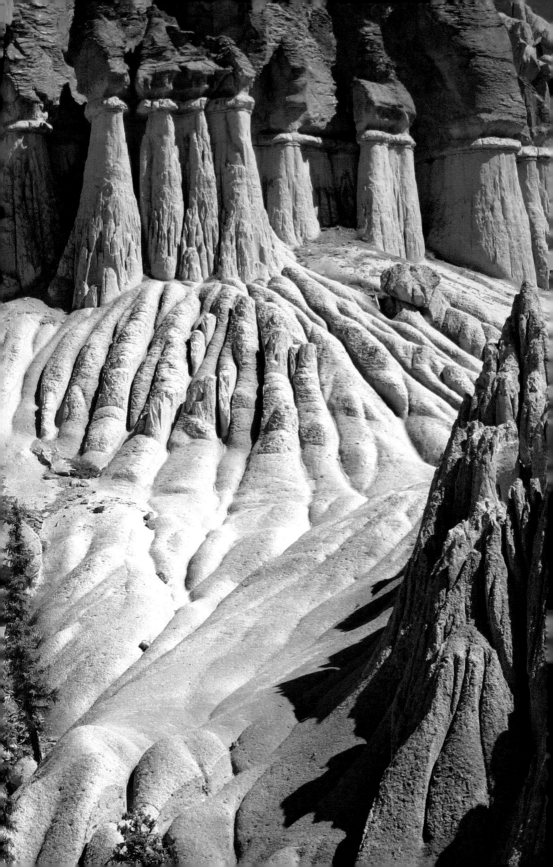

# WHEELER GEOLOGIC AREA

## 46

**Directions:** From Creede, drive 7³/₁₀ miles southeast on Highway 149 to Pool Table Road #600 (Spring Gulch). Turn north and travel approximately 10 miles. You'll come to the remains of Hanson's Sawmill. Park here (there is a 4WD track that continues on from here but don't attempt it without <u>very high clearance</u> and not in wet weather). From Hanson's Sawmill, a 6⁴/₅ mile hike (one-way) will bring you to the Wilderness boundary. From there, a 3¹/₅ mile loop takes you through the area. Due to the length of the hike and the altitude (10,000'+) an overnight visit is highly recommended. Bring ample water!

**Contact Info:**
Rio Grande National Forest
719-852-5941
www.fs.fed.us/r2/riogrande
www.sangres.com/features/wheelergeologic.htm

**Fee:** no fee

**Hours:** always open—but do it when there's some daylight

**Best time to visit:** anytime you can get there is a good time to be there; but try to avoid the heat of mid-summer

**Camping/Lodging:** basic camping on forest land just outside wilderness boundary; nearest lodging in Creede

**Access:** the road to Hanson's Sawmill is good; the hike from there is moderate to difficult, especially because of the altitude

**Jon's Rating:** ★★★★☆ (geology)

**Jon's Notes:**
Thirty million years ago was not a good year for Creede. About that time, someone unwittingly irritated La Garita volcano and it showed displeasure by throwing a mega-volcanic fit. Mountains of ash and volcanic tuff were blown into the sky by the explosion, blanketing the area for miles around. Now here we are, a few years later, having to deal with the mess. And what a fine mess it is! Wheeler Geologic Area is an incredible collection of erosional features reminiscent of the Badlands of South Dakota, only much more dramatic.

*LEFT: This area is a dynamic erosional landscape of spires and pinnacles which are especially attractive to space aliens and Elvis impersonators.*

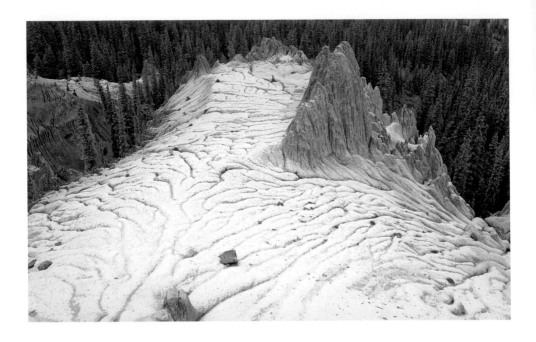

*The culprit of all this distortion of reality is selective weathering, a nifty geologic term that can be thrown around at parties once you learn what it means.*

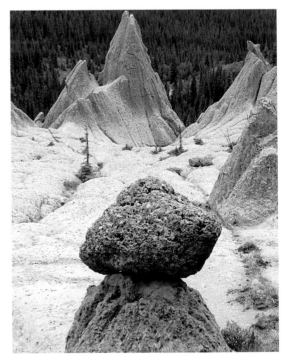

## NO MORE NATIONAL MONUMENT

It's hard to imagine, but this was Colorado's first national monument. It was originally granted National Monument status in 1908 by Teddy Roosevelt. Along about 1950, the feds determined it was too remote and costly to create access roads so the property lost its monument status and was transferred to the Forest Service. Funds were cut and the roads quickly fell into disrepair. The Forest Service christened it Wheeler Geologic Area and then incorporated it into the La Garita Wilderness Area when that was formed.

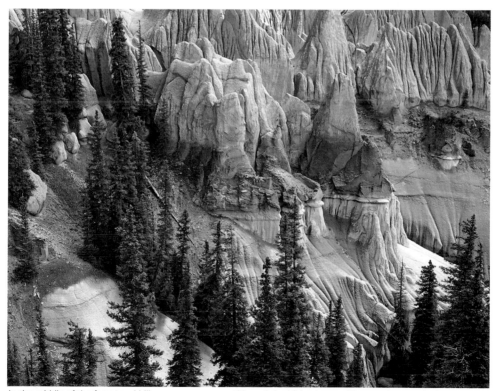

*In the middle of the forest and hills you come across this weird sci-fi landscape. It's surreal to say the least.*

## Museums

### The Anasazi Heritage Center

www.co.blm.gov/ahc/index.htm
27501 Highway 184
Dolores, Colorado 81323
970-882-5600

The Anasazi Heritage Center is a federal museum, research center, and curation facility that introduces visitors to Four Corners prehistory. Approximately three million records, samples, and artifacts from public lands throughout southwestern Colorado form the Center's holdings. The Heritage Center is also the visitor center for the new Canyons of the Ancients National Monument, with fantastic exhibits and informational displays. Visit this facility before you go to the ruins.

### Denver Museum of Nature and Science

www.dmns.org
2001 Colorado Blvd.
Denver, CO 80205
303-322-7009

The Denver Museum of Nature & Science is the Rocky Mountain region's leading natural history museum with some of the finest paleontology and archaeology exhibits in the country. A variety of exhibitions, programs, and activities help Museum visitors experience the natural wonders of Colorado, Earth, and the universe.

### Dinosaur Journey

www.dinosaurjourney.org
550 Jurassic Court
Fruita, CO 81521
970-858-7282

This museum was once in jeopardy of closing down altogether but now it's in good hands and fulfilling its mission. The Museum of Western Colorado's Dinosaur Journey is in Fruita, Colorado, right in the heart of dinosaur country. It features the latest exhibits and information about dinosaurs of western Colorado, eastern Utah and surrounding areas. It also has realistic robotic dinosaurs and a working paleontology laboratory.

## Dinosaur Ridge Museum

**www.dinoridge.org**
16831 W. Alameda Pkwy
Morrison, CO, 80465
303-697-3466

The Dinosaur Ridge area is one of the world's most famous dinosaur fossil localities. Here, in 1877, some of the best-known dinosaurs were first discovered. In 1989, the Friends of Dinosaur Ridge formed to address increasing concerns regarding the preservation of the site and to offer educational programming on the area's resources. Today, Dinosaur Ridge is a destination for over 70,000 dinosaur enthusiasts, students of all ages, and nature aficionados each year.

## Koshare Indian Museum

**www.koshare.org/contact/**
115 West 18th Street
La Junta, CO 81050
719-384-4411

"Koshare" is not a tribe but rather a character portrayed in dances in many Pueblo Indian cultures. Don't let the name fool you, this museum houses an impressive collection of Southwestern artifacts, mostly from Pueblo tribes.

## Louden-Henritze Archaeology Museum

**www.santafetrailscenicandhistoricbyway.org/lharcmus.html**
Frudenthal Memorial Library
Trinidad State Junior College
Trinidad, Colorado 81082
719-846-5508

The Trinidad State Jr. College Archaeology Department was established in 1942. Throughout the years, many noted archaeologists have taught at the college and conducted excavations and scientific studies at numerous sites in the region. They recorded many finds, recovered artifacts during supervised excavations, and cataloged and stored the artifacts at the college. This museum is their legacy.

## The Morrison Natural History Museum

501 Colorado Highway 8
Morrison, CO 80465
303-697-1873

Morrison is the namesake of the original dinosaur discoveries in the Denver area. The Morrison Natural History Museum's combination of personal, hands-on tours in the relaxed, rustic atmosphere of a small foothills cabin creates a unique experience with every visit. Here you explore the life and landscapes of west Denver for the past 150 million years.

## Rocky Mountain Dinosaur Resource Center

**www.rmdrc.com**
201 S. Fairview St.
Woodland Park, CO  80863
719-686-1820

Sometimes things are just done better by private enterprise. This admirable institution is the result of years of effort and planning by Mike and JJ Triebold, two very enthusiastic paleo professionals. Located on the main drag of Woodland Park, this museum features over 12,000 square feet of paleontology exhibits, focusing on dinosaurs and other Mesozoic fossils—most of which are excavated and prepared exclusively by the center. Go see it!

## University of Colorado Museum

**http://cumuseum.colorado.edu**
CU Museum, UCB 218
University of Colorado
Boulder, Colorado  80309
303-492-6892

With more than four million artifacts and specimens, the CU Museum houses one of the most extensive and respected natural history collections in the Rocky Mountain and Plains regions, making it one of the top university natural science museums in the country.

# The Ute Indian Museum

**www.visitmontrose.net/indian_museum.htm**
1519 E. Main St.
Montrose, CO  81402
800-873-0244

One of the few museums in the country devoted solely to one tribe; the Ute People were the indigenous inhabitants of western Colorado. The museum commemorates their life and culture and is located on the farm once belonging to the famous Ute leader, Ouray, and his wife, Chipeta.

# References

Bostwick, Todd W., 2002, Landscape of the Spirits, University of Colorado Press, Tucson, CO

Chronic, Halka, 1980, Roadside Geology of Colorado, Mountain Press Publishing, Missoula, MT

Cunkle, James R. and Jacquemain, Markus A., 1996, Stone Magic of the Ancients, Golden West Publishers, Phoenix, CO

Ferguson, William M. and Rohn, Arthur H., 1990, Anasazi Ruins of the Southwest in Color, University of New Mexico Press, Albuquerque, NM

Frazier, Deborah, 2000, Colorado's Hot Springs, Pruette Publishing Company, Boulder, CO

Knopper, Steve, 2006, Moon Handbooks–Colorado, 6th edition, Avalon Travel Publishing, Emeryville, CA

Noble, David Grant, 2000, Ancient Ruins of the Southwest, Northland Publishing, Flagstaff, CO

Malotki, Ekkehart and Weaver, Donald E., 2002, Stone Chisel and Yucca Brush, Kiva Publishing, Walnut, CA

McCreery, Patricia and Malotki, Ekkehart, 1994, Tapamveni, Petrified Forest Museum Association, Petrified Forest, CO

## Websites

**Government websites:**
www.nps.gov
www.fs.fed.us
www.co.blm.gov
www.fs.fed.us/r2/recreation/Heritage/index.shtml
www2.nature.nps.gov

**Other non-commercial websites:**
www.greatmuseums.org/colorado.html
www.centerfordesertarchaeology.org
www.americansouthwest.net/Colorado
www.hikingincolorado.org

**Commercial websites:**
http://rockart.esmartweb.com
www.sidecanyon.com

# GLOSSARY

**anthropomorph** OK, I admit this sounds a bit out there but here goes: Anthropomorphs are rock art images which resemble human forms, at least a little. Some folks think they're more likely space aliens which could account for the many strange appendages and ornamentations often found within these images. Not to mention the sudden disappearance of guidebook authors at such sites.

**archaeoastronomy** It's apparent that ancient peoples had a pretty good grasp of celestial goings-on. The archaeologists who became interested in studying these things decided they needed a title for their new science, and preferred one that was a good tongue twister.

**archaeology** Why are you asking me this? You should know it already! It's basically the study of ancient cultures, their remains, artifacts, structures, and influences.

**Archaic** In North America, the native cultures which predate the ancestral pueblo peoples (Hisatsinom) but occur after Clovis time. The Archaic period is roughly defined as running from about 6,000 BC to about 900 BC.

**basalt** It's old lava—simple as that.

**Clovis** Primarily refers to a distinct form of stone tool manufacturing. Clovis points are fundamentally more refined and advanced than previously fabricated tools. The term also, more loosely, defines cultures that fall within a temporal context after PaleoIndians but predating Archaic. Generally considered from about 10,000–6,000 years BC.

**Cocci** aka "Valley Fever," Abbreviation of the medical term Coccidioidomycosis, a not-very-enjoyable lung disease endemic to the Southwest. Something you will want to avoid.

**desert patina/desert varnish** The effect is as if some cosmic woodworker spilled a very large bucket of dark stain over the desert floor, coating all the exposed rock on the surface. That stain is comprised mostly of iron oxides that color the outer surface dark brown to black, while the inside is the natural rock color, usually much lighter.

**dike/dyke** A geologic descriptor for igneous material which intrudes into other rocks in a more-or-less vertical orientation. If the surrounding rock is softer and erodes away, the dyke sticks up, often forming sharp ridges.

**erg** An uncommon but useful geologic term describing any vast land area covered with sand and sand dunes.

**eye** Here I take the easy way out and pull that old dictionary trick by telling you to go look up the term "window" which, lucky for you, actually is defined on page 219.

**geoglyph** A singularly cool archeological site made by either aligning/piling rocks into designs and shapes, or, alternatively, by deliberate removal of stones from an area creating recognizable patterns in the ground during the process.

**geology** A very cool and hip career if you can make a living at it, which most geology graduates have a hard time doing, myself included. The term refers to the study of the Earth and the processes that continue to shape it.

**hard-rock** No, it's not a cafe. OK, so it IS a cafe, but that has nothing to do with what we're talking about here. In this case it's a geology and mining term referring mostly to metamorphic and igneous rock

**Hephaestus** The ancient Greek god of fire, son of Zeus and Hera. Probably not someone you'd want to tick off.

**Hisatsinom** A somewhat loosely-defined group which primarily refers to ancestral Hopi. The Hisatsinom had their start as a recognizable group about 900 BC, just after the Archaic.

**hog-back** Another one of those trite geologic terms coined by some drunken Scotsman who thought he saw some semblance of animal physiology in a pile of rocks that stood on end.

**igneous** Rock which forms more-or-less directly from a molten state. As opposed to ignoramus—a person which is headed in such a way.

**lava** You should know this already, but here's a little more info for ya: Yes, we all know this is volcanic in origin. But lava need not have come from a stereotypical volcano. It often arrives by out-pouring from large cracks in the Earth's crust.

**lava tube** A natural tunnel that forms when a lava "river" exits from a channel in the lava flow.

**lithology** Refers to rock, and I don't mean rock-and-roll bands. Rather it's all about stony rock—the different types, their composition, and the processes that produce them. Also can mean the subdivision of geology which studies rock.

**magma** Molten rock or lava before it has cooled. Don't tangle with this stuff.

**metamorphic** A classification of rock which forms by subjecting parent rock to intense heat and pressure thereby altering its chemistry without completely melting it. Sort of like what happens to parents as they raise kids.

**metate** Stone grinding surface used by native cultures to pulverize corn and other plant material.

**PaleoIndian** Term given to all ancestral Indians that predate well-documented dominant native cultures. In North America this generally refers to any pre-Clovis peoples older than about 8,000 years.

**paleontology** The study of fossils, which, in turn, has nothing to do with the watch-making company of the same name.

**paper shales** On rare occasion, some shales have such extremely fine laminae, they literally split into layers no heavier than the thickness of a sheet of paper. In such cases where fossils occur they are often preserved in exquisite detail. Florissant Fossil Beds is well known in this regard.

**pegmatite** Another nebulous geologic term which loosely defines a diverse group of coarse-crystal granites that are high in quartz and feldspar and often occur in veins or dikes. If you suspect you've got some on your property, you'll be happy to know they're also a good place to look for gold.

**petroglyph** Petro means rock, glyph means form. Can you add them and come up with something other than "rock form?" This term also references the way in which the image is made—etched or inscribed into the rock face by pecking away the outer surface.

**pictograph** Meaningful painting on rocks by ancient cultures. (As opposed to meaningless painting on subway cars, which we scientists call "graffiti.")

**pueblo** Do I really need to spell this out for you? OK, OK it's a term used to denote a communal building structure that generally houses multiple families and is the center of activity for a given community.

**riparian** Has nothing to do with repairing anything. Refers to natural environments that abide along permanent waterways. Home to wildlife galore.

**sedimentary** My sentiments about sediments: They're pretty cool rocks which form as accumulations of particles from the breakdown of other rocks.

**selective weathering/selective erosion** The key here is "selective"—like "selective service" when Uncle Sam calls you up for military duty. Certain rocks are softer than others and erode away much faster, leaving the harder, more durable, rock to stand out like a Marine Special Forces recruit in a monastery.

**sink** If you're thinking of the catchment basins in your house then you're not too far off. Now imagine a depression in the ground which effectively performs similarly to your kitchen sink and you've got it.

**soft-rock** We are not referring to elevator music or "smooth jazz" here. The sedimentary rock to which this term applies is usually not as hard as its counter-parts in the metamorphic or igneous realm. So if it comes to throws, bet on the hard-rock—it'll kick soft-rock's butt every time.

**strata** Another fancy geology term used to confound unsuspecting party-goers. Basically refers to layers of rock.

**tree-ring dating** You're probably astute enough to know this phrase isn't hinting at a romantic night out between two annular growths of tall woody plants. But what you may not know is it refers to an absolute method of dating ruins which contain preserved tree parts in their structure. By looking at the patterns in the annular rings, researchers are often able to match them precisely with known records of tree growth, thereby pinpointing the years the tree was alive.

**troglodyte** Don't take it personally, but if you are fairly primitive and like to live in seclusion—especially in a cave—then you're a troglodyte. But it's not all bad. You probably don't have to pay for air-conditioning, do you?

**volcanic bomb** It's not something likely to turn up in Transportation Safety Administration (TSA) checks of luggage at the airports, but you never know. When a volcano explodes and hurls liquid magma skyward, the globs cool and harden as they fly through the air, developing tell-tale shapes before hitting the ground or clueless bystanders.

**window** If you had a solid wall on your house that you wanted to let the sun shine through, what would you do? Smash a hole in the sucker, of course. That bit of handiwork is called a window. Now let me ask you, why should Mother Nature shy away from doing the same thing when she wants to have sunlight stream through a hard rock wall?

# INDEX

# ALSO AVAILABLE

If you enjoyed the *Colorado Journey Guide,* you'll also want to check out the *Arizona Journey Guide and the New Mexico Journey Guide.* With similar formats and all of the same great features, these journey guides are perfect for residents, tourists and snowbirds alike. Explore the 60 best spots in the Grand Canyon State and the 49 top locales in the Land of Enchantment, and make it a visit to the Southwest that you'll never forget!

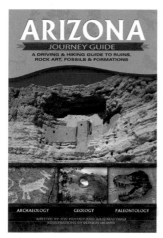

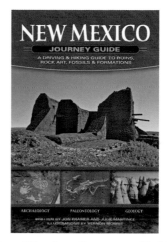

**Arizona Journey Guide**
*272 pages • 6" x 9" • softcover*
*$16.95 • ISBN: 978-1-59193-140-9*

**New Mexico Journey Guide**
*232 pages • 6" x 9" • softcover*
*$16.95 • ISBN: 978-1-59193-221-5*

# ABOUT THE AUTHORS

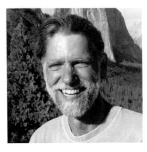

**Jon Kramer** is an adventurer first, and also a geologist, writer, climber and surfer (but not necessarily in that order, depending on the surf). He received his Bachelor of Science degree in geology at the University of Maryland and has pursued life as an adventuring paleontologist ever since. His interests are quite varied and include all things natural. In addition to popular travel and adventure writing, Jon has published scientific papers on critters as ancient as 2 billion-year-old bacteria and as young as 12,000-year-old mammoths. Jon travels extensively with his wife Julie, sometimes settling down for a rest in Minnesota, Florida, California and interesting points in between.

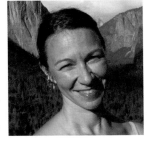

**Julie Martinez** is an explorer, naturalist, freelance artist and formal art instructor. Her appreciation for insects, plants, rocks and fossils started in childhood with a collection that has grown throughout her life. Julie graduated from the University of Wisconsin, Stevens Point, with a degree in Fine Arts and Biology. She initially worked as an illustrator for the medical field but in the late 1980s began a freelance career, which she has enjoyed ever since. Julie's work is featured in many textbooks, journals and museum exhibits throughout North America. She is also a staff teacher at Minnesota School of Botanical Art. When not teaching, she travels with Jon, exploring the wilds of the world.

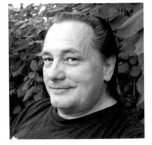

**Vernon Morris** is a freelance artist, muralist and adventuring time traveler. His formal art education took place in the early 1980s at the University of Minnesota and Minneapolis College of Art and Design. Vern's Native American (Anishinabe) roots have been a powerful influence in his life. He maintains a small quarry at Pipestone National Monument where he excavates the famous carving stone every year. He then sculpts it into pipes and ritual objects just as his ancestors did for countless generations. Vern carries his work with him into the wilds and is just as comfortable carving pipestone atop a mesa in the Southwest as sketching scenes from antiquity along the ocean in Big Sur.